AF869126

Hopefully this
a beautiful, gentle &
effective medicine
more real to you!

much Love –

Oriental Medicine & You:

Making a Seemingly Complex 3,500-year-old Medicine Understandable for the Layperson

Curry D. Chaudoir,
Diplomate in Acupuncture

500 W. Silver Spring Drive, Suite #K205
Glendale, WI 53217

ISBN# 978-0-615-45636-2

Library of Congress Control Number: 2011905620

The statements in this book have not been evaluated by the Food and Drug Administration. The information in this book is for educational purposes only. Nothing in this document is intended as a substitute for your doctor's diagnosis and/or treatment. If you suspect you have a medical problem, seek competent medical help. Neither the author nor the publisher shall have any liability to any person or entity with regard to claims, loss, injury, or damage caused, or alleged to be caused, directly or indirectly by the use of information contained herein, or damage arising from any information or suggestion in this book.

Printed at Malloy Incorporated, Ann Arbor, MI

Dedication

This book is for the millions of patients who have suffered with seemingly unexplainable conditions, been given incomprehensible diagnoses and little or no options for help.

Foreword

Communicating with patients, in a way that clearly explains how Acupuncture and Herbal Medicine work and how they help specific health concerns, is vital to the success of a practitioner. It is just this type of communication that Curry so magnificently brings across in his everyday practice and with this wonderful book.

More and more, the practice of medicine in this country is becoming integrated. The divide is narrowing gradually between Western and Eastern Medicine, this being the heart of the reason why we must, as practitioners and as members of the health care community, pay more attention. Not only to our own standards of education, but to adequate means of patient education and health care awareness as well.

This book serves as an important tool that can help practitioners and patients reach this goal. It elegantly simplifies, translates, and merges Chinese Medicine concepts with modern biomedical conditions that are prevalent in health care today.

Whether you are a practitioner, student or patient, I believe you will find this text to be an invaluable resource in your pursuit for knowledge, health, and well-being.

Tina Chen, Licensed Acupuncturist
President, Evergreen Herbs and Medical Supply, LLC

Acknowledgements

Oriental Medicine and You would have been impossible without the help and insight of many friends and family members. My wife, the beautiful April, offered incredible support throughout the creation of this book. My immediate family--Mom, Molly, Eva, Justin, Katherine, Mom, Dad--inspired me every step of the way. Special thanks to the Acupuncture and Holistic Health Associates team for their contributions: Laura Patiño for her editing, typesetting and image contributions, Amanda Iglinski for her graphic design insights, Amber Martin for her editing expertise, Mary Netzer for her work on image placement and content input, Jennifer Fekete, Sara Carter, Morgan Davis, Gretel Weiskopf, Scott Martin, and David Fife. I am very grateful to the ancient and contemporary physicians of Oriental Medicine who breathed life into this beautiful medicine and my practice; in particular Dr. Jiang Zheng, Dr. Giovanni Maciocia, Dr. Jimmy Chang, Dr. Richard Tan, Dr. John Chen and Tina Chen. Thank you to Dr. David Singer for the continual, exuberant inspiration. I am grateful to every patient we ever had the honor of helping. And finally, thanks to numerous family and friends who continue to offer support and assistance-you know who you are; it means more than you can imagine.

About This Book

This book's purpose is to make Oriental Medicine, *the people's medicine*, accessible to the reader. Over the past several thousand years, Oriental Medicine has developed into the most comprehensive medical system on the planet, initially passed on via oral tradition and then written word. This work is a humble translation of ancient Chinese medical theory into layman's contemporary English terminology.

This work is not a complex text laden with medical terminology for use by medical and/or scientific academics who scour materials in search of what *doesn't* work; rather it is a work based upon: 1. the truths of Oriental Medicine as outlined in many texts used to train Acupuncture professionals, and 2. experience with 1000's of patients and *their* reality.

This book is intended as a reference for use by:

- Patients curious about Acupuncture and Oriental Medicine, and/or
- Acupuncturists who would like to offer their patients an understandable explanation of their particular symptom(s) prior to beginning care.

It is recommended you read the following introduction, Chapter One and Chapter Two, all of which give insight into the eloquent beauty, effectiveness and simplicity of this ancient medical tradition. Then refer to the alphabetical list of specific medical conditions and their solutions in Chapter Three. Use this guide for a better understanding of various ailments and their correction from the Oriental Medicine perspective.

I love hearing from my readers at *curry@milwaukeeacu.com* or find me at http://www.facebook.com/cchaudoir.

Introduction

This is a manual designed to help you, the reader, understand the theory of Oriental Medicine as it relates to your individual condition. Oriental Medicine--which includes the use of exercise, nutrition, Acupuncture, Chinese herbs and massage--has been in development for thousands of years. Although the medicine may seem complex, it is truly simple to understand if one adopts the logical, basic concepts regarding the simplicity and reality of the body. This manual is designed to make this seemingly complex medicine quite simple. Understanding the true nature of your condition is an essential first step toward resolving the condition.

In my experience with thousands of patients, I have seen that there are four main areas where Oriental Medicine distinguishes itself from conventional Western Medicine:

1. In conventional Western Medicine the symptom alone is diagnosed and treated; in Oriental Medicine the underlying cause of a person's symptom is diagnosed and treated to resolve the symptom.

2. In conventional Western Medicine, the *quantities* of bodily substances (for example, the number of Liver enzymes in the blood stream) and images of the body's internal parts (for example, those images viewed via X-ray or MRI) are the most important diagnostic tools used; in Oriental Medicine, *qualities* and relationships between systems in the body are the most important diagnostic tools used. The following illustrates this difference: an Acupuncturist may observe--using the diagnostic tools of Oriental Medicine to understand the relationships between bodily

systems--that mental stress decreases Liver function, causing the Liver to negatively affect the Heart, which may constrict the blood vessels, in turn leading to high blood pressure. In contrast, a Medical Doctor may check one's blood pressure using the systolic and diastolic quantities given, to simply indicate that "stress" causes high blood pressure without understanding *why* the high blood pressure exists, only that the *symptom* of high blood pressure exists.

3. Conventional Western Medicine is unsurpassed in the diagnosis of health problems; however, it is often unable to effectively resolve chronic conditions. Conventional Western Medicine is most useful in the treatment of acute, crisis situations, whereas Oriental Medicine is excellent in the diagnosis and treatment of long-term, chronic problems. Additionally, many acute conditions may benefit from immediate Oriental Medical treatment, for example ankle sprains and the like heal rapidly if treated in the first two weeks following the injury.

4. Conventional Western Medicine views the body as static and unchanging; Oriental Medicine views the body as dynamic and capable of change in many ways. For example, it is common for a Medical Doctor to say, "You have diabetes and you'll have to live with it." An Acupuncturist may say, "Let's improve Spleen/Pancreatic system function so that the body utilizes more of its own insulin to improve the diabetes."

The following is a look at the body *as it is* from the point of view of Oriental Medicine. It is recommended you read Chapter One, then fill out the survey in the beginning of Chapter Two and use the main text of the book as a reference, not necessarily reading cover-to-cover.

Ideally, the treatment of a medical condition focuses on the *underlying cause* of a health concern rather than merely addressing the symptom. To eliminate a symptom and its cause, partnership with professionals who utilize functional Acupuncture and/or Chinese Medicine is essential.

Table of Contents

Chapter 1:	Oriental Medicine Basics	12
	The Five Branches of Oriental Medicine	13
	The Organ System	14
	The Circulatory System	19
Chapter 2:	Using Oriental Medicine to Find out about Yourself	23
	Five Element Survey	24
Chapter 3:	The Conditions	25
	Abdominal Gas and Bloating	26
	Acid reflux and Heartburn	28
	Acne	30
	Allergies to Airborne Particles	32
	Allergies to Food	34
	Anemia	36
	Angering Easily	37
	Anxiety	39
	Arthritis	41
	Asthma	43
	ADD/ ADHD	45
	Bell's Palsy	47
	Blood Pressure Problems	50
	Bursitis	53
	Cancer	54
	Carpal Tunnel	56
	Cholesterol Problems	58
	Constipation	60
	Depression	62
	Diabetes	64
	Digestive Problems- General	66
	Diarrhea	68
	Diverticulitis	70
	Dizziness and Vertigo	71
	Endometriosis	73
	Eye Problems (Dry Eyes, Itchy Eyes, Gritty Eyes, Blurry Vision, Floaters, Double Vision, Visual Disturbances, Ocular Migraines, Etc.)	75
	Fatigue	77
	Fibromyalgia	79
	Fluid Metabolism and Distribution Problems	81
	Foot/Ankle Problems	83
	Frustration	84
	Hair Loss	87
	Headaches	89
	Hemorrhoids	91
	High Blood Pressure	92
	Hot Flashes	95
	Hypothyroid (under-active thyroid)/ Hyperthyroid (over-active thyroid)	96
	Impotence	98
	Incontinence- Bowel	100
	Incontinence- Urinary	102
	Infertility- Men	103
	Infertility- Women	105
	Insomnia- Difficulty Fall Asleep	107
	Insomnia- Waking in the Middle of the Night	109
	Insomnia- Waking up Early in the Morning	111
	Irritability	113
	Irritable Bowel Syndrome	116
	Low Blood Pressure	118

Memory: Long-Term Memory Loss 120
Memory: Short-Term Memory Loss 121
Menopausal Hot Flashes 122
Menopausal Insomnia- Difficulty Falling Asleep 124
Menopausal Insomnia- Waking at Night 126
Menopausal insomnia- Waking Early 128
Menopausal Mood Swings 130
Menopausal Night Sweats 132
Menopausal Vaginal Dryness 134
Menstrual Clotting 136
Menstrual Cramping 138
Migraines 140
Mood Swings 142
Muscle Cramping 144
Narcolepsy 145
Neuropathy 148
Night sweats/ Heat in the Body at Night 150
Osteoporosis 152
Pain Due to Scar Tissue 153
Pain: Lower Back 155
Pain: Neck, Shoulder, and Elbow 157
Pain: Upper Back, Lower Back, Arm, Leg, Joints 159
Parkinson's Disease 161
Pre-Menstrual Cramping 163
Pre-Menstrual Digestive Problems 165
Pre-Menstrual Mood Swings 168
Post-Stroke Syndrome 171
Prostate Problems 173
Restless Leg Syndrome 174
Ringing in the Ears 176
Sciatica/ Hip Pain 178
Shingles 180
Sinus Problems 182
Skin Conditions 185
Smoking Cessation 187
Snoring 188
Spinal Column Disk Problems 191
Spinal Stenosis 193
Stress, Difficulty Adapting to 195
Tendonitis 198
Thyroid Imbalances 199
TMJ Syndrome 201
Tremors 203
Varicose Veins 205
Weight Problems 206
Wrist Pain 208
Image Credits 210
Recommended Reading 212
Find a Practitioner Near You 213
About the Author 214
Index 215

Chapter 1:

Oriental Medicine Basics

Given that Oriental Medicine has been developing for thousands of years, it is inevitable that many schools of thought have developed various viewpoints regarding the body, reasons for functional decline, reasons for symptoms onset and treatment of those symptoms. Fundamentally, however, there are basic principles that are agreed upon by most, if not all, practitioners of Oriental Medicine.

THE FIVE MAIN BRANCHES OF ORIENTAL MEDICINE

The ancient physicians of Oriental Medicine discovered that use of at least the following methods of care from birth onwards would give the greatest chance of living happily and healthily to 120 years of age.

1. "Right Thinking," which includes all forms of exercise, both ancient and contemporary.

2. Oriental Nutrition, which encourages the use of certain foods dependent on the individual's body type and the season.

3. Acupuncture, which involves the insertion of fine, stainless steel needles into specific points on the body to restore circulation and thus, function.

4. Chinese Herbal Medicine, which utilizes many plant and mineral substances in combination to restore circulation and function.

5. Massage, which involves manipulation of tissues of the body to encourage function and circulation.

These five branches have been used for thousands of years to restore function to two fundamental body systems that govern overall health: the organ system and the circulatory system, both of which we will now discuss.

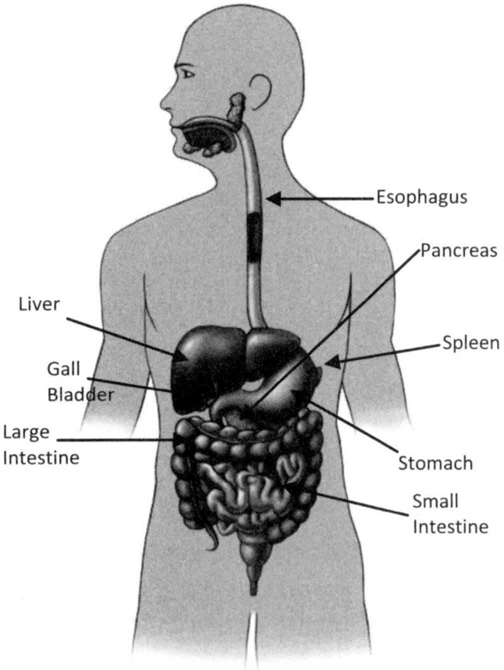

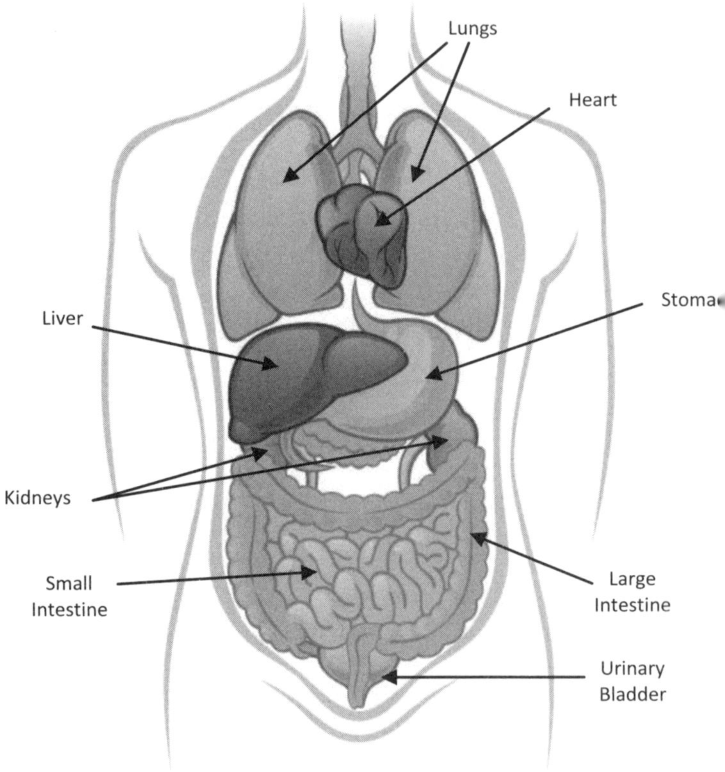

THE ORGAN SYSTEM

The body's organ system (see diagrams above) in Oriental Medicine comprises the glandular system, the Lungs, the Large Intestine, the Stomach, the Spleen/Pancreatic system, the Liver, the Gall Bladder, the Heart, the Small Intestine, the Pericardium (the tissue surrounding the Heart), the Kidney/Adrenal system, the Urinary Bladder, and an organ network known as the "Sanjiao" (English translation: "three burner," which describes three distinct organ systems that together regulate body temperature, water distribution and digestion).

The organ system is closely linked with glandular function. For example, the Spleen and Pancreas are anatomically connected; when an Acupuncturist discusses "Spleen" function, he/she is actually referring to the Spleen/Pancreatic system which produces insulin that allows the body to utilize sugars, stimulates immune system function, produces certain blood cells, assists the Stomach in metabolism of food and facilitates nutrient distribution throughout the body via the bloodstream. Another commonly misunderstood organ/gland relationship is the Kidney/Adrenal system. When an Acupuncturist uses the term "Kidney," the reference is made to both the Kidneys and the Adrenal glands, which are anatomically connected. The Kidney/Adrenal system produces crucial raw materials for hormone production. For example, the Kidney/Adrenal system stimulates the pituitary gland which in turn releases thyroid stimulating hormone to the thyroid which affects the bones, growth, development, metabolism, body temperature and Heart rate.

Clinically, it is quite clear that function governs structure, not the other way around. Examples discovered in Oriental Medicine of organs governing specific body structures follow: the Spleen/Pancreatic system governs the production and density of muscle tissue; the Kidney/Adrenal system governs the production and density of bone tissue, the spine, bone marrow, brain tissue and the nervous system; and the Liver governs the tendons and ligaments.

What follows are the body's main organs' *dynamic* functions from Oriental Medicine's view point[1], which are quite extensive when compared to conventional Western Medical theory. Links to the emotions are discussed in the following descriptions; keep in mind physicians in China began to explore the nature of human emotion thousands of years ago and discovered a direct relationship between human emotion and the organ system.

One should note that all of the following functions occur only when the organ is *healthy* and functions *optimally*.

---

[1] Maciocia, Giovanni, *The Foundations of Chinese Medicine*, New York: Churchhill Livingstone, 1989. 498p.

The Heart governs the blood, controls the blood vessels, shows its health in the complexion, houses the mental faculties of the individual (the Heart, in fact, is referred to as the "king" of emotions), opens to the tongue and controls perspiration.

The Liver--among its 600 functions--"stores" the blood, ensures free circulation of blood and energy throughout the body, controls the tendons and ligaments, shows its health in the fingernails and toenails, opens into the eyes and is said to influence one's ability to plan and find direction in life.

The Lungs govern energy/oxygen/respiration, control the blood vessels and circulation, "disperse" and "descend" (meaning they send oxygen and fluids taken from the air into the bloodstream), regulate water passageways, control the skin, control the hair, are related to the body's movement and encourage sharp, clear sensory function.

The Spleen/Pancreatic system governs the "transformation" and "transportation" of food and fluids throughout the body; controls blood; controls the muscles; controls the arms and legs; opens to the mouth; shows its health in the lips; "suspends" the organs and other tissues in their correct location and is said to influence thinking, studying, concentrating, focusing and memorizing.

The Kidney/Adrenal system is connected with one's genetic line, governs birth, governs growth, governs reproduction, governs development, produces the "marrow," nourishes the brain, controls the bone tissue, governs water and fluid distribution throughout the body, assists oxygen distribution throughout the body, opens into the ears, shows its health in the hair, controls the opening and closing of the anus and urethra and is said to influence one's ability to focus on goals and pursue them effectively.

The Pericardium, a sac of tissue surrounding and protecting the Heart, shares the Heart's functions and is said to influence one's relations with others.

The Stomach (closely associated with Spleen/Pancreatic system function) "ferments" the food and drink one consumes thus making it usable by the body, helps transport the nutrients from food throughout the body, moves the food and fluids downward into and through the digestive tract and is said to be the "origin" of the vital fluids of the body.

The Small Intestine receives and transforms further the mostly digested food and fluid from the Stomach; it also separates usable from unusable fluids, sends unusable fluids to the Urinary Bladder and is said to influence one's ability to distinguish important from unimportant life issues.

The Large Intestine receives digested foods and fluids from the Small Intestine, re-absorbs some of those fluids and excretes the stools.

The Gall Bladder stores bile that is produced by the Liver, excretes bile upon consumption of fats and is said to influence one's ability to make decisions.

The Urinary Bladder transforms, stores and excretes fluids.

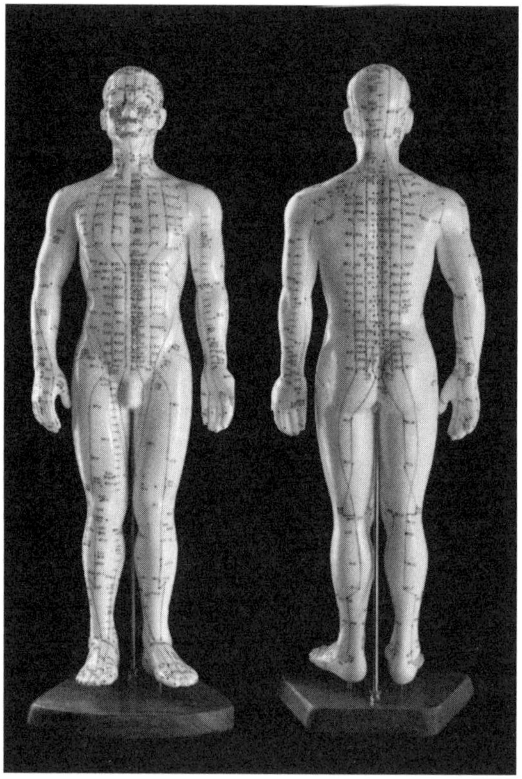

Closely linked and perhaps inseparable from the organ system is a popular concept in Oriental Medicine known as the "meridian system" (see diagram above). The "meridian system" refers to pathways in the body--taken from the concept of lines on a globe--which is perceived to be a system distinct and separate from the blood vessels, the nerves, and the lymphatic system. It is said to circulate "Qi" (pronounced "chee", this Chinese term most easily translates as "energy" or "vital force") that originates in each organ and travels on specific pathways on both sides of the body. Qi is said to be similar to electricity, however may have far more complex and interesting properties than electricity.

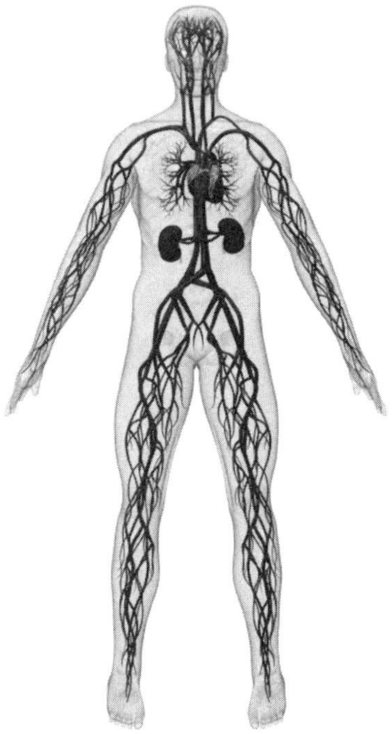

THE CIRCULATORY SYSTEM

The second fundamental system governing overall body function is the circulatory system (see diagram above) which includes the veins, arteries, and capillaries (the smallest of blood vessels) that carry blood (filled with nutrients, hormones and oxygen) between the Heart and every single cell. The initial building blocks of blood, derived from the bone marrow, are supplemented via digestive organ transformation of food and fluids into much smaller, usable nutrients. These nutrients then pass through the intestine wall into the bloodstream, thereby creating the volume of blood necessary for overall body function.

These two systems discussed above, the organs and circulation, obviously overlap; when functioning normally they promote ideal health. When either system is out of harmony, is not functioning properly, or is overwhelmed by outside stressors, the body will break down and symptoms will develop over time.

The typical decline from health to chronic symptoms follows: one is born with optimal function, however, as one goes through life is exposed to three potential stressors: mental/emotional, environmental/chemical (preservatives in food, poor air quality, etc.) or physical. Those stresses accumulate over time and the body breaks down, eventually losing function and developing "incorrect" habit patterns known as the disease process (example: asymptomatic diabetes). Finally, the body will exhibit symptoms (in the case of diabetes, abnormal glucose levels, dry mouth, neuropathy, etc.). The symptom is the *final* stage of the breakdown; remarkably, in most cases a symptom is not present unless that area of the body is functioning at less than 40% of normal. The symptom is the last stage of the decline of the body and it is the first thing to disappear under care.

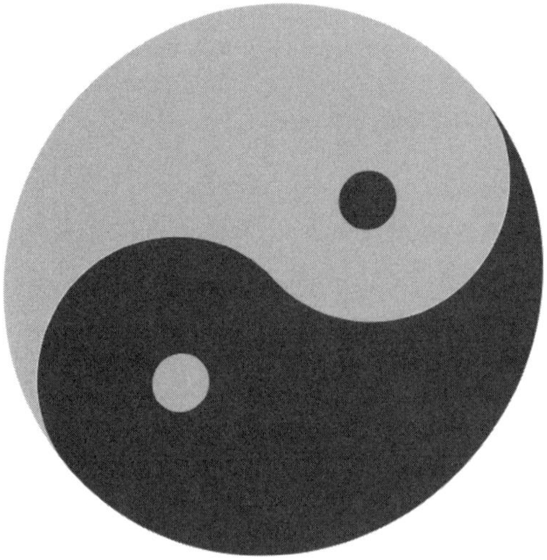

Another basic and very important Oriental Medical theory is that of yin and yang (see diagram above), two interrelated and interdependent concepts used to describe relationships between things in the natural world. Yin (a Chinese term translated literally as "the shady side of the mountain") refers to those aspects in the body which are cool, moist, still and nourishing. One example of yin is the fluid that protects and surrounds the baby in a mother's womb. Yang (a Chinese term translated literally as "the sunny side of the mountain") refers to those aspects in the body which are hot, dry, invigorating and moving. One example of yang is the incredibly active process of transforming food in the digestive system into usable nutrients and their delivery to every cell in the body. Yin and yang are said to both exist simultaneously to a greater or lesser degree in each organ; similarly a person's entire body, although composed of yin and yang may tend to be more yin or more yang, dependent on several factors such as genetics and/or lifestyle. For example, someone who seems "to always feel hot and dislike summer" is said to have more yang relative to yin than someone who seems "to always feel cold and dislike winter."

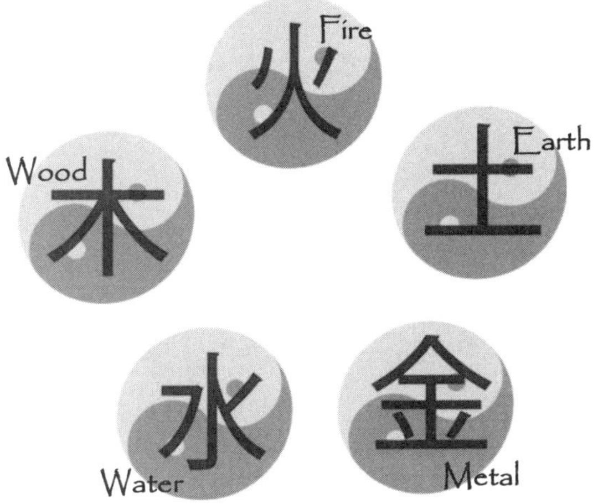

Another very important concept in Oriental Medicine is Five Element theory (see diagram above), which describes basic elements (fire, earth, metal, water, and wood) in the body and the inter-relationships of those elements similar to those same elements found in nature. Each element corresponds to specific organs, flavors, emotions, colors, seasons, etc. One such element is fire, which corresponds to the Heart, Small Intestine, Pericardium, and Sanjiao ("Sanjiao theory" is discussed above) function. Another element is earth, which corresponds to Spleen/Pancreatic system and Stomach function. The metal element corresponds to Lung and Large Intestine function. The water element corresponds to Kidney/ Adrenal system and Urinary Bladder function. The wood element corresponds to Liver and Gallbladder function.

Please take the survey in the following section to understand more about potential imbalances in each of your main organ systems as they relate to the Five Elements.

Chapter 2

Using Oriental Medicine to find out about Yourself

Please fill out the following survey by marking all of the items that apply to you. The purpose of this survey is to determine which organs are potentially in need of treatment. Then you can reference the main section of this book immediately after the survey, which elaborates upon the underlying causes of individual health problems. Ideally, if the Five Elements were harmoniously balanced and the body healthy, one would have none of the following symptoms. If one or more symptoms exist, it indicates a likely imbalance in the indicated organ system below.

Five Elements Survey: Check all that apply to you. (The following list is not exhaustive.)

Water Element

Items marked in this section indicate Kidney/Adrenal system and Urinary Bladder imbalances

__ Trouble sleeping/ insomnia
__ Sore knees
__ Weak Knees
__ Low back pain
__ Body temperature problems
__ Night sweats
__ Heat in the hands, feet, and chest
__ Hot flashes any time of the day
__ Thirsty
__ Swollen feet
__ Frequent cavities
__ Easily broken bones
__ Memory problems
__ Excessive hair loss
__ Low-pitched ringing in the ears
__ Kidney stones
__ Bladder infections
__ Wake during the night twice or more to urinate
__ Lack of bladder control
__ Fear
__ Easily startled

Wood Element

Items marked in this section indicate Liver and Gall Bladder imbalances

__ Migraines/ headaches
__ Neck pain/ tension
__ Shoulder pain/ tension
__ Mood swings
__ Tight sensation in the chest
__ Bitter taste in the mouth
__ Anger easily
__ Frustration
__ Depression
__ Irritability
__ Unable to adapt to stress
__ Headache
__ Lump in the throat
__ Hip pain
__ High-pitched ringing in the ears
__ Eye and vision problems

Earth Element

Items marked in this section indicate Spleen/Pancreas and Stomach imbalances

__ Abdominal bloating and gas
__ Gurgling noise in the Stomach
__ Fatigue after eating
__ Easily bruised
__ Hemorrhoids
__ Over-thinking
__ Worry
__ Low Appetite
__ Digestive irregularities (constipation, diarrhea, etc.)
__ Sensation of heaviness in the body
__ Mental heaviness/ sluggishness/ fogginess
__ Nausea
__ Fatigue
__ Bad breath
__ Bleeding, swollen, or painful gums
__ Acid regurgitation
__ Belching
__ Hiccoughs
__ Stomach pain
__ Vomiting

Fire Element

Items marked in this section indicate Heart, Small Intestine and Pericardium imbalances

__ Palpitations
__ Anxiety
__ Sores on the tip of the tongue
__ Restlessness
__ Mental confusion
__ Chest pain traveling to shoulder
__ Frequent dreams
__ Swollen hands

Metal Element

Items marked in this section indicate Lung and Large Intestine imbalances

__ Allergies
__ Sinus Problems
__ Cough
__ Dry skin
__ Sneezing
__ Sore throat
__ Difficulty breathing
__ Sadness

Chapter 3

The Conditions

Note: The following list is not exhaustive; rather, it represents commonly treated conditions in modern Acupuncture clinics.

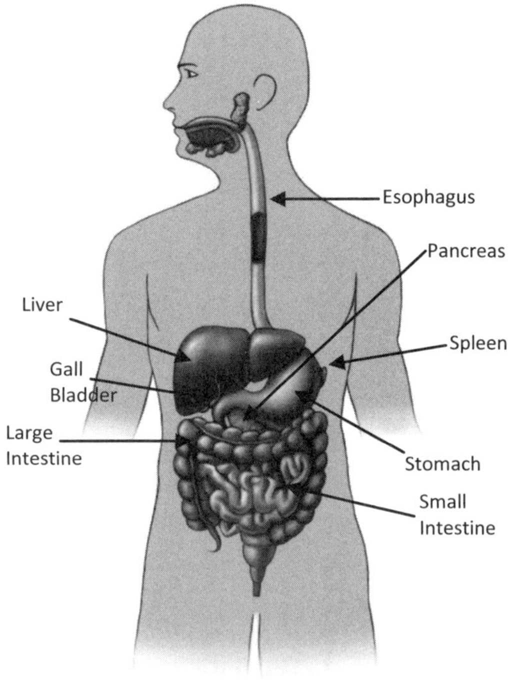

Abdominal Gas & Bloating

Abdominal gas and bloating have many potential causes, however what follows are the basic mechanics. The Spleen/Pancreatic system is in charge of making sure the food you put into your Stomach is broken down into small nutrients and are distributed in the blood stream to create blood and energy. If the Spleen/Pancreatic system is not functioning efficiently it can cause a problem with the food not fully being broken down, which leads to bloating and/or abdominal gas.

The Kidney/Adrenal system, which provides the "spark" for Spleen/Pancreatic system function, is another possible source of gas and bloating.

The following is a useful analogy: the Kidney/Adrenal system is the digestive system's "pilot light" and the Stomach is the "cauldron" in which food is placed and "heated" by the Spleen/Pancreatic system, which is the “burner” upon which the pot is placed to cook the food. If any of these parts of the digestive process falter, it leads to inefficient metabolism, possibly leading to abdominal gas and/or bloating.

As you can see with this particular health problem, there is an underlying cause. The key to success in treating these problems lies in addressing the underlying issue described above to eliminate the problem over the long term. To speed Acupuncture and/or Chinese Herbal Medicine results, it is recommended one minimally reduce or eliminate the intake of caffeine, dairy, deep-fried foods, sugar, preservatives in food, chemicals in food, raw vegetables and municipal tap water (which most often contains chlorine and fluoride, considered by many as dangerous chemicals).

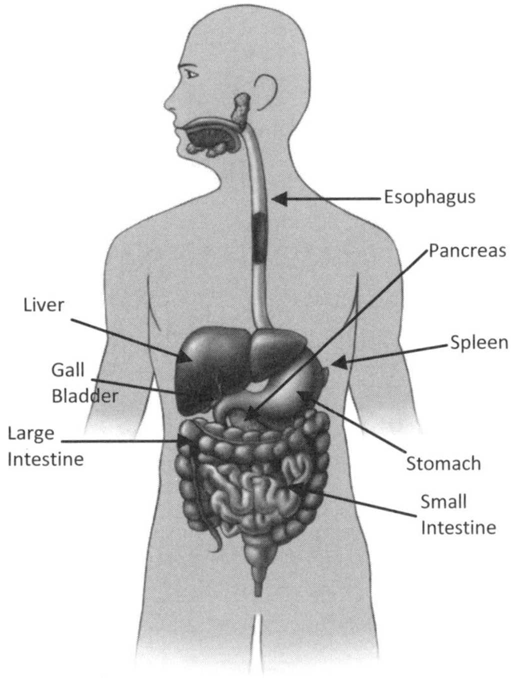

Acid Reflux & Heartburn

Acid reflux and Heartburn have multiple potential causes, however what follows are the basic mechanics. Although other organs (such as the Liver) may be involved, the Stomach is often directly related to acid reflux and Heartburn, as its general purpose is to move things such as food and fluid downward upon eating. When one eats, food is supposed to travel downward through the esophagus and into the Stomach. The food is then supposed to pass through the Stomach *downward* into the intestinal tract. A loss of Stomach function may cause acid to flow upwards, resulting in pain and discomfort. In Oriental Medicine this is referred to as "rebellious flow of the Stomach" meaning substances flow in the reverse direction the body intends. In some cases, it may also happen that the Stomach produces too much acid for various reasons causing an overflow of acid upwards into the esophagus.

As you can see with this particular health problem, there is an underlying cause. The key to success in treating these problems lies in addressing the underlying issue described above to eliminate the problem over the long term. To speed Acupuncture and/or Chinese Herbal Medicine results, it is recommended one minimally reduce or eliminate the intake of caffeine, deep-fried foods, sugar, preservatives in food, chemicals in food and municipal tap water (which most often contains chlorine and fluoride, considered by many as dangerous chemicals).

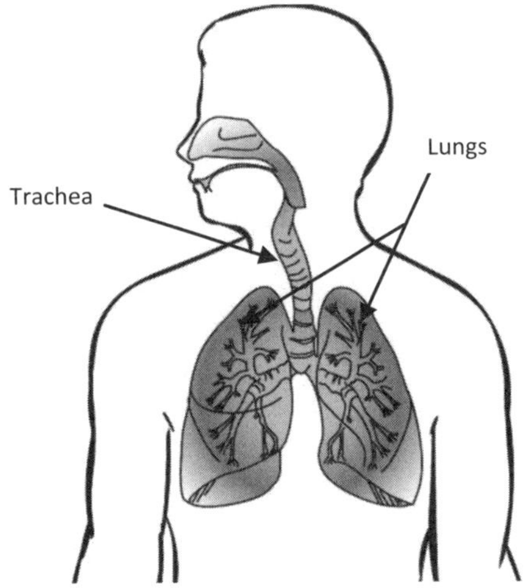

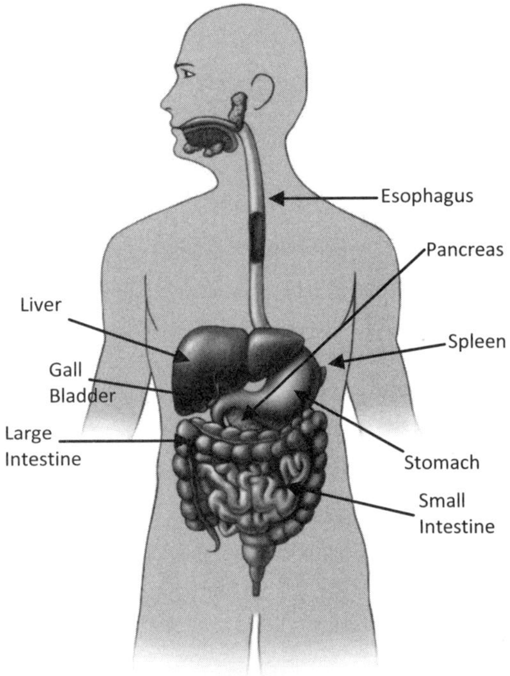

Acne

Acne has many potential causes, however what follows are the basic mechanics. The Lungs and the Liver govern the skin's function. If the Lung and/or Liver malfunction the body may ineffectively attempt to eliminate accumulated toxins from the organ system and/or the fatty tissue via the skin, often on the face and/or back. In Oriental Medicine this is, in many cases, referred to as "Hot Above/Cold Below," indicating that "heat" (inflammation and toxicity) are rising to the surface of the body, agitating the skin. Simultaneously, "cold" "sinks" into the lower organ system, including the Large Intestine, Small Intestine, Kidneys, Urinary Bladder, etc., which explains why many acne sufferers have impaired digestive function. Conversely, some people may have an excess of heat and inflammation which cause the acne.

As you can see with this particular health problem, there is an underlying cause. The key to success in treating these problems lies in addressing the underlying issue described above to eliminate the problem over the long term. To speed Acupuncture and/or Chinese Herbal Medicine results, it is recommended one minimally reduce or eliminate the intake of caffeine, deep-fried foods, dairy, sugar,

preservatives in food, chemicals in food and municipal tap water (which most often contains chlorine and fluoride, considered by many as dangerous chemicals).

Given that one of the Liver's 600 functions is to purify the bloodstream, reducing or eliminating the intake of toxic chemicals is very important as part of a larger strategy to resolve acne. It is also important to exercise vigorously (to a point of perspiration) for at least 30 minutes four times weekly, thus increasing Liver circulation, soothing the Liver and stimulating increased circulation throughout the body, which allows the body to detoxify most effectively.

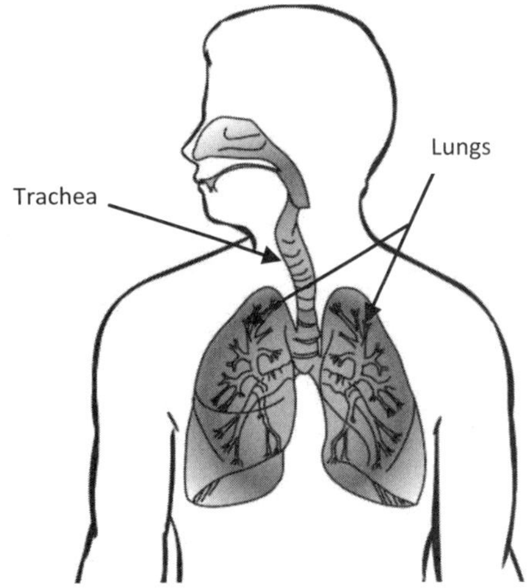

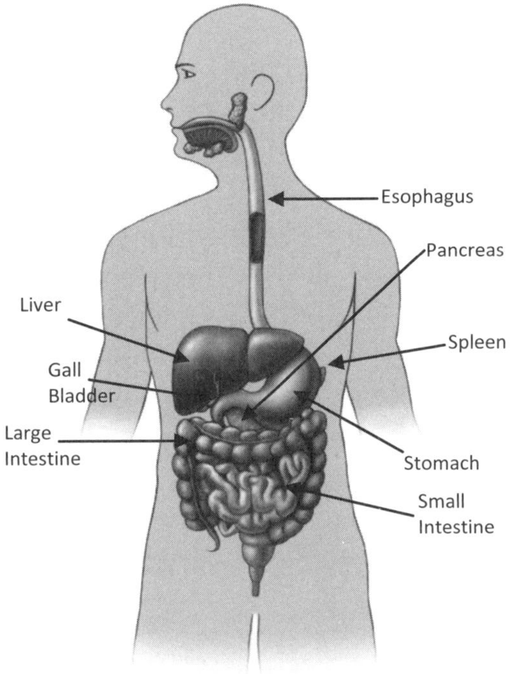

Allergies to Airborne Particles

Allergies have many potential causes, with variations from person to person, however what follows are the basic mechanics. The Spleen and the Lungs govern the immune system; although other systems in the body may be involved, these are most common culprits.

The Spleen, understood in Western Medicine as part of the lymphatic system, governs internal immune function. The lymphatic system eliminates unnecessary and unhealthy material such as toxins and pathogens from the body. The following is a useful analogy: the lymphatic system could be likened to the alley behind a city home where debris is removed, whereas the circulatory system could be likened to the street in front of the house through which groceries and other needed items enter.

Spleen function generates internal immune system activity, fighting pathogens that penetrate deeper into the body and destroying pathogens in the blood stream to prevent internal allergies. If one were to eat or inhale a potential allergen, a well-functioning Spleen eliminates such material.

The Lungs, which open to the nose, throat, and sinuses, govern external immune function. If the sinuses and the Lungs are functioning well, the nasal mucosal membranes carry immune system factors that destroy incoming pathogenic material such as pollen.

The following 2,000-year-old Chinese Medical quote helps to clarify further these organs role in immune function: *when the Spleen malfunctions it may cause fluids to accumulate in the body; when the Lungs malfunction they will take on those fluids.* An example illustrating this principle follows: one consumes food and fluids that the Stomach and Spleen cannot fully metabolize. Those fluids may "travel" upwards into the Lungs. The Lungs, to protect themselves, may activate the cilia (very fine hairs designed to move substances upwards out of the Lungs), which may likely push the fluids into the sinuses, causing sinus problems.

As you can see with this particular health problem, there is an underlying cause. The key to success in treating these problems lies in addressing the underlying issue described above to eliminate the problem over the long term. To speed Acupuncture and/or Chinese Herbal Medicine results, it is recommended one minimally reduce or eliminate the intake of caffeine, deep-fried foods, dairy, sugar, preservatives in food, chemicals in food and municipal tap water (which most often contains chlorine and fluoride, considered by many as dangerous chemicals).

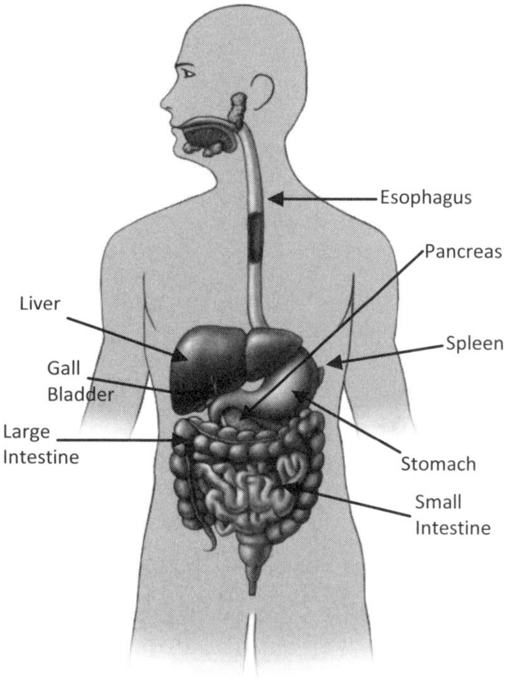

Allergies to food

Allergies have many potential causes, with variations from person to person, however what follows are the basic mechanics. The Spleen and the Lungs govern the immune system; although other systems in the body may be involved, these are most common culprits.

The Spleen, understood in Western Medicine as connected to the lymphatic system, governs internal immune function. The lymphatic system eliminates unnecessary and unhealthy material such as toxins and pathogens from the body. The following is a useful analogy: the lymphatic system could be likened to the alley behind a city home where debris is removed, whereas the circulatory system could be likened to the street in front of the house through which groceries and other needed items enter.

Spleen function generates internal immune system activity, fighting pathogens that penetrate deeper into the body and destroying pathogens in the blood stream to prevent internal allergies. If one were to eat or inhale a potential allergen, a well-functioning Spleen eliminates such material.

As you can see with this particular health problem, there is an underlying cause. The key to success in treating these problems lies in addressing the underlying issue described above to eliminate the problem over the long term. To speed Acupuncture and/or Chinese Herbal Medicine results, it is recommended one minimally reduce or eliminate the intake of caffeine, deep-fried foods, dairy, sugar, preservatives in food, chemicals in food and municipal tap water (which most often contains chlorine and fluoride, considered by many as dangerous chemicals).

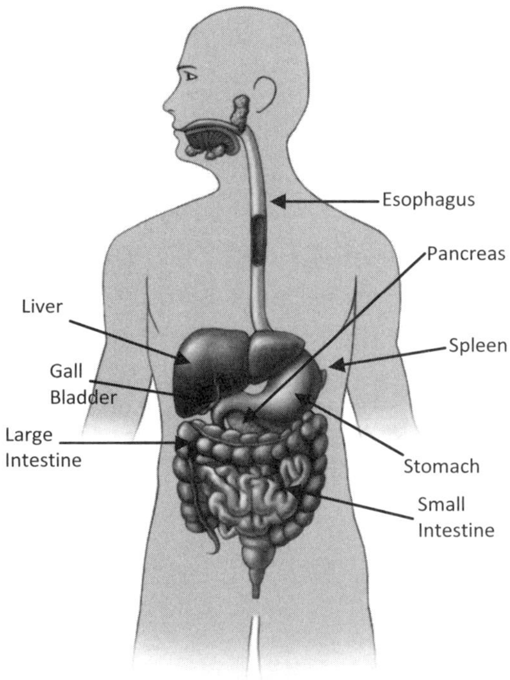

Anemia

Anemia has many potential causes, however what follows are the basic mechanics. One of the Spleen/Pancreatic system's primary functions is to "transform" (break down) food into usable nutrients, including iron, and to "transport" (distribute) those nutrients throughout the body via the blood stream. Lack of Spleen/Pancreatic function can lead to iron deficiency (anemia).

As you can see with this particular health problem, there is an underlying cause. The key to success in treating these problems lies in addressing the underlying issue described above to eliminate the problem over the long term. To speed Acupuncture and/or Chinese Herbal Medicine results, it is recommended one minimally reduce or eliminate the intake of caffeine, deep-fried foods, dairy, sugar, preservatives in food, chemicals in food and municipal tap water (which most often contains chlorine and fluoride, considered by many as dangerous chemicals).

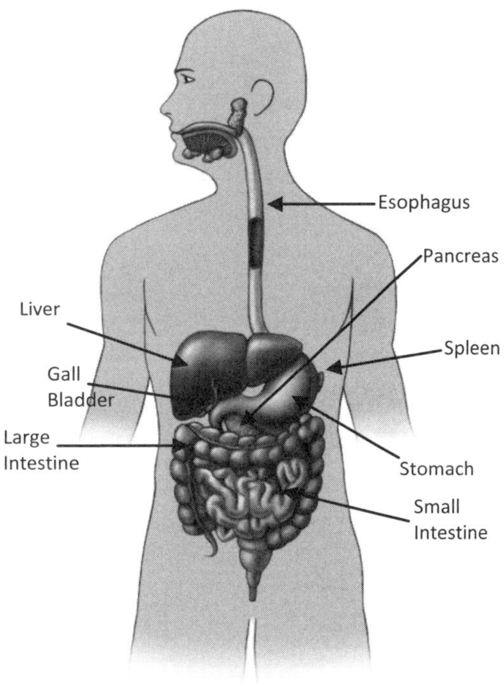

Angering Easily

There are many reasons one may consistently anger easily (without particular cause), however what follows are the basic mechanics. Thousands of years ago, physicians in China began to explore the nature of human emotion and discovered a direct link between emotion and the organ system. Having helped many people resolve emotional imbalances over the years, we've found the following to be accurate from the point of view of the physical body (obviously many factors exist in life that may trigger bodily malfunction which, in turn, could then trigger an emotional response). What is described below is the relationship between the emotions and physical body.

The Liver has 600 physiological functions, one of which is to help the body adapt to the mental and emotional stresses of life. In other words, if one's Liver is functioning at a high level, stress entering one's life has no physical effect; however, if one's Liver isn't functioning well, stress can have a negative effect on the body.

Liver malfunction can cause a person to experience excessive or inappropriate anger, irritability, frustration, impatience, and/or depression. For example, a person with multiple emotional stresses over many years may experience suppressed Liver function. Then, the loss of a loved one could cause Liver function to drop dramatically, and the person could then begin to anger easily without apparent cause. On the other hand, a well-functioning Liver will cause one to be emotionally even.

Angering easily can be caused by a breakdown in Liver function, not simply an imbalance in brain chemistry (the typical Western Medical view of this particular condition). Ironically, addressing only the brain chemistry with medication often leads to further difficulty resolving the problem as shown here: if one takes a medication for angering easily (which may be caused by a Liver imbalance) and that medication reduces Liver function (the Liver, in its capacity as a blood purifier, will attempt to eliminate the chemical from the body), it makes it more difficult to treat the anger. This explains why a person may take a medication their entire life... and angering easily never fully resolves!

Given that one of the Liver's 600 functions is to purify the bloodstream, reducing or eliminating the intake of toxic chemicals is very important as part of a larger strategy to resolve angering easily. It is also important to exercise vigorously (to a point of perspiration) for at least 30 minutes four times weekly, thus increasing Liver circulation, soothing the Liver and stimulating increased circulation throughout the body, which allows the body to detoxify at least to a small degree.

As you can see with this particular health problem, there is an underlying cause. The key to success in treating these problems lies in addressing the underlying issue described above to eliminate the problem over the long term. To speed Acupuncture and/or Chinese Herbal Medicine results, it is recommended one minimally reduce or eliminate the intake of caffeine, deep-fried foods, dairy, sugar, preservatives in food, chemicals in food and municipal tap water (which most often contains chlorine and fluoride, considered by many as dangerous chemicals).

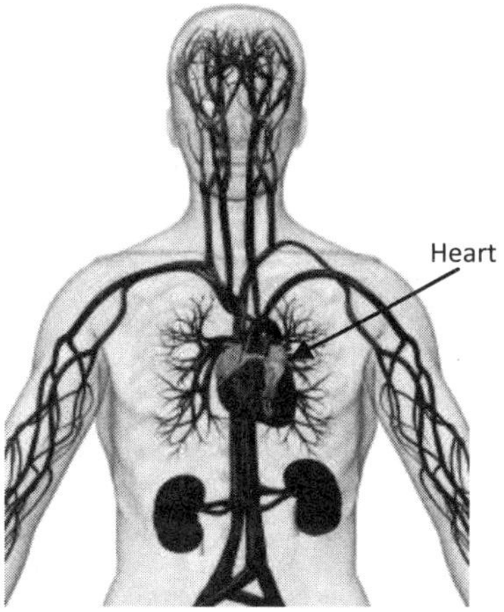

Anxiety

There are many reasons one may experience anxiety, however what follows are the basic mechanics. Thousands of years ago, physicians in China began to explore the nature of human emotion and discovered a direct link between emotion and the organ system. Having helped many people resolve emotional imbalances over the years, we've found the following to be accurate from the point of view of the physical body (obviously many factors exist in life that may trigger bodily malfunction which, in turn, could then trigger an emotional response). What is described below is the relationship between the emotions and physical body.

In Oriental Medicine the Heart is known as the "king" of emotions; an imbalance in Heart function may cause a person to experience many problems including anxiety and/or panic attacks. It has been discovered that a breakdown in Heart function will cause one to tend toward anxious feelings or panic attacks. One can see the correlation clearly: a panic attack is often accompanied by a repetitive, intense perceptible heartbeat (known as "palpitations").

As you can see with this particular health problem, there is an underlying cause. The key to success in treating these problems lies in addressing the underlying issue described above to eliminate the

problem over the long term. To speed Acupuncture and/or Chinese Herbal Medicine results, it is recommended one minimally reduce or eliminate the intake of caffeine, deep-fried foods, dairy, sugar, preservatives in food, chemicals in food and municipal tap water (which most often contains chlorine and fluoride, considered by many as dangerous chemicals).

Arthritis

Arthritis has many potential causes, however what follows are the basic mechanics. Western Medicine offers two classes of arthritis: *rheumatoid arthritis* and *osteoarthritis*. Rheumatoid arthritis (usually involving inflammation) is diagnosed when certain cells are present in the blood stream and osteoarthritis (usually involving joint breakdown) is diagnosed when there is joint deterioration.

Oriental Medicine offers more distinct classifications including twelve categories of "arthritic" problems. The term "Bi" (pronounced "bee" and translated to mean "obstruction" or "blockage") is a Chinese term used to denote arthritic conditions. There are twelve categories of "Bi" syndromes (the word "syndrome" indicates the overall make-up of a health problem). A "Wind-Bi" syndrome is one classification of pain that moves around in the body. Obviously this classification of "wind" is purely symbolic; the pain, in this case, "moves around in the body like the wind." This particular diagnosis does not imply wind exists in the body; rather it describes the pain pattern.

Other "Bi" syndrome classifications involve moisture (referred to as a "Damp-Bi" syndrome), heat (referred to as a "Hot-Bi" syndrome), cold (referred to as a "Cold-Bi" syndrome), etc....all of which may lodge in the muscles and/or joints, causing decreased circulation, decreased energy circulation, pain, inflammation and/or swelling.

Often such a condition may develop as such: one experiences a physical trauma--such as a car accident--which causes tissue damage and subsequent scar tissue. The injured area then becomes susceptible to one or more outside climatic factors, such as moisture. Years later, the person is able to "tell you when it's going to rain" due to the moisture lodged in the injured area causing pain.

As you can see with this particular health problem, there is an underlying cause. The key to success in treating these problems lies in addressing the underlying issue described above to eliminate the problem over the long term. To speed Acupuncture and/or Chinese Herbal Medicine results, it is recommended one minimally reduce or eliminate the intake of caffeine, deep-fried foods, dairy, sugar, preservatives in food, chemicals in food and municipal tap water (which most often contains chlorine and fluoride, considered by many as dangerous chemicals).

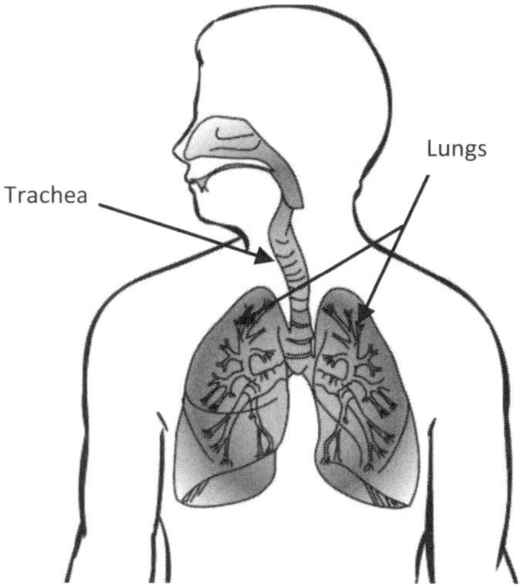

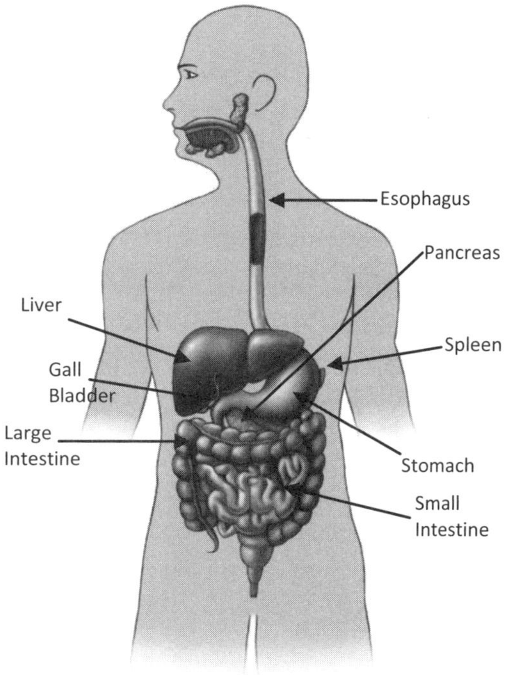

Asthma

Asthma has many potential causes, however what follows are the basic mechanics. Although other systems in the body may be involved, the organs most often related to asthma are the Spleen and the Lungs as they are vital to fluid distribution.

The following 2,000-year-old quote helps to clarify further these organs role in immune function: *when the Spleen malfunctions it may cause fluids to accumulate in the body; when the Lungs malfunction they will take on those fluids.* An example illustrating this follows: one consumes food and fluids that that the Stomach and Spleen cannot fully metabolize. Those fluids may "travel" upwards into the Lungs. The Lungs, to protect themselves, may activate the cilia (very fine hairs designed to move substances upwards out of the Lungs), which may likely push those fluids out of the Lungs and out of the body via the sinuses. If the cilia are not functioning properly or if the cilia are rendered useless because too much fluid congests the Lungs, it may cause a spasm, experienced as a cough or wheezing.

As you can see with this particular health problem, there is an underlying cause. The key to success in treating these problems lies in addressing the underlying issue described above to eliminate the problem over the long term. To speed Acupuncture and/or Chinese Herbal Medicine results, it is recommended one minimally reduce or eliminate the intake of caffeine, deep-fried foods, dairy, sugar, preservatives in food, chemicals in food and municipal tap water (which most often contains chlorine and fluoride, considered by many as dangerous chemicals).

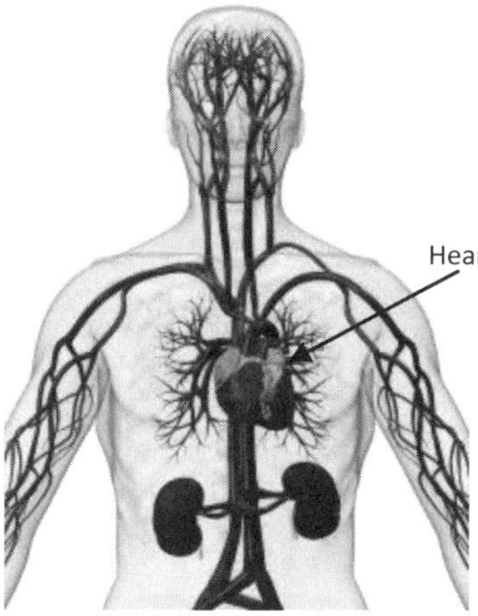

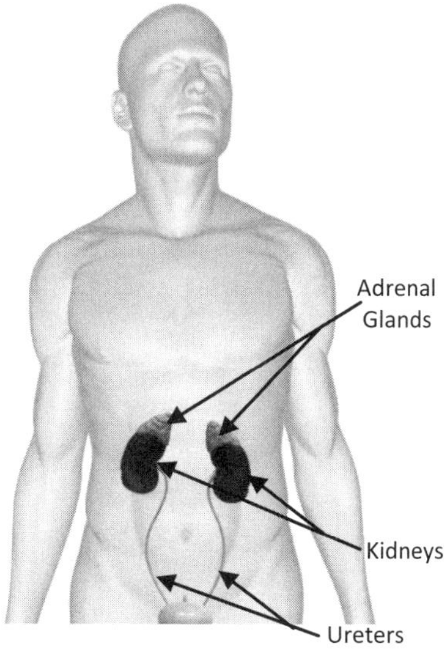

Attention Deficit Disorder (ADD)/ Attention Deficit Hyperactivity Disorder (ADHD)

Attention Deficit Disorder and Attention Deficit Hyperactivity Disorder have many potential causes, however what follows are the basic mechanics at work. It is said that the Heart "governs" the function of the mind (the mental capacity of the individual).

Inability to focus and/or concentrate is often caused by a loss of Heart function, wherein the mind becomes over-stimulated. On the other hand, restlessness may be due to a Kidney/Adrenal imbalance that causes the body to be overactive at inopportune times (i.e. when a child is sitting in class).

If one takes a medication for such conditions, and that medication reduces Liver function, it may make it more difficult to treat the condition.

As you can see with this particular health problem, there is an underlying cause. The key to success in treating these problems lies in addressing the underlying issue described above to eliminate the problem over the long term. To speed Acupuncture and/or Chinese Herbal Medicine results, it is recommended one minimally reduce or eliminate the intake of caffeine, deep-fried foods, dairy, sugar, preservatives in food, chemicals in food and municipal tap water (which most often contains chlorine and fluoride, considered by many as dangerous chemicals).

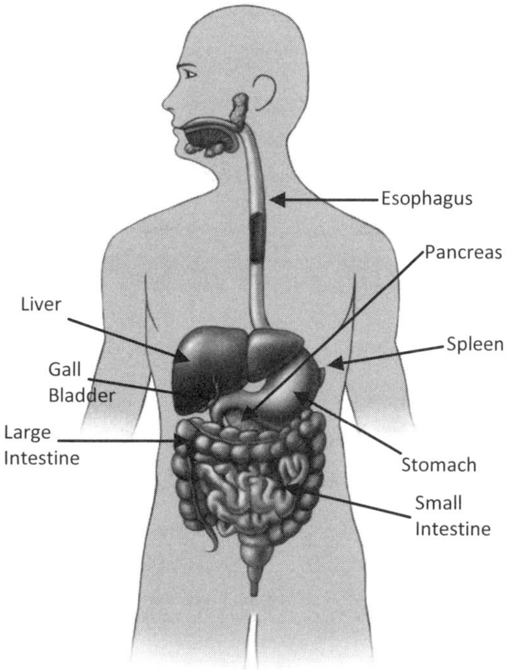

Bell's Palsy

Bell's Palsy has several potential causes, however what follows are the basic mechanics causing the associated facial droop, numbness, tingling and/or discomfort.

What follows are three possible causes of Bell's Palsy (one or more may be present to trigger an episode).

1. Exposure to significant amounts of wind with a weakened immune system: it is common, for example, in gusty Shanghai, China for bicyclists exposed to the wind to experience Bell's Palsy. The muscles and nerves in the affected area are actually "attacked" by the wind, leading to the symptoms described above.

2. A breakdown in Liver function: as one of its 600 functions, the Liver is responsible for helping one adapt to the mental and emotional stresses of life. Loss of Liver function may reduce the individual's ability to handle stress, which overwhelms the body and may disrupt the Gall Bladder,

which, in turn, obstructs circulation to the facial muscles and nerves, causing Bell's Palsy.

3. Nervous system malfunction: stresses may build up over a period of time, overloading the body and causing a "short circuit" where the muscles and nerves of the face completely malfunction, leading to Bell's Palsy.

The following is an example of an actual female patient where all three factors described above were involved: a gas station manager was under extraordinary emotional stress for some time, which caused a decline in Liver and nervous system function. Then, in a windy 1996 snowstorm, she ran in and out of the gas station several times without a jacket or a scarf to shovel snow. The next day, she woke with her face numb and drooping on the left side.

We have discovered that Bell's Palsy responds best to treatment immediately after onset. It is, of course, possible to resolve the problem after one has had the problem for a long time; however, recovery generally takes proportionately longer.

A Bell's Palsy Prevention Tip: wear a scarf to protect your neck in windy conditions.

Given that one of the Liver's 600 functions is to purify the bloodstream, reducing or eliminating the intake of toxic chemicals is very important as part of a larger strategy to treat and/ or prevent Bell's Palsy. It is also important to exercise vigorously (to a point of perspiration) for at least 30 minutes four times weekly, thus increasing Liver circulation, soothing the Liver and stimulating increased circulation throughout the body, which allows the body to detoxify at least to a small degree.

As you can see with this particular health problem, there is an underlying cause. The key to success in treating these problems lies in addressing the underlying issue described above to eliminate the

problem over the long term. To speed Acupuncture and/or Chinese Herbal Medicine results, it is recommended one minimally reduce or eliminate the intake of caffeine, deep-fried foods, dairy, sugar, preservatives in food, chemicals in food and municipal tap water (which most often contains chlorine and fluoride, considered by many as dangerous chemicals).

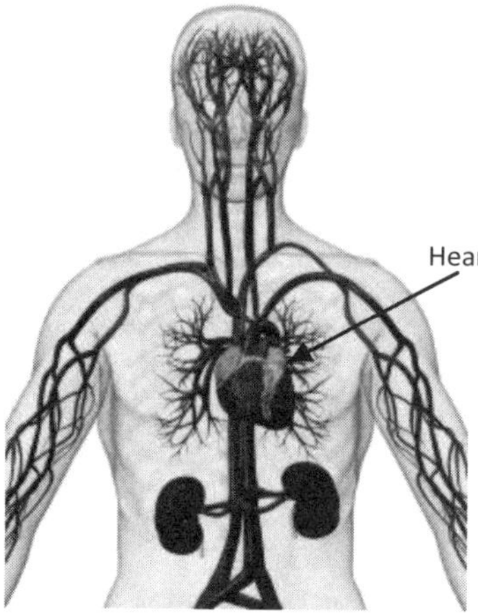

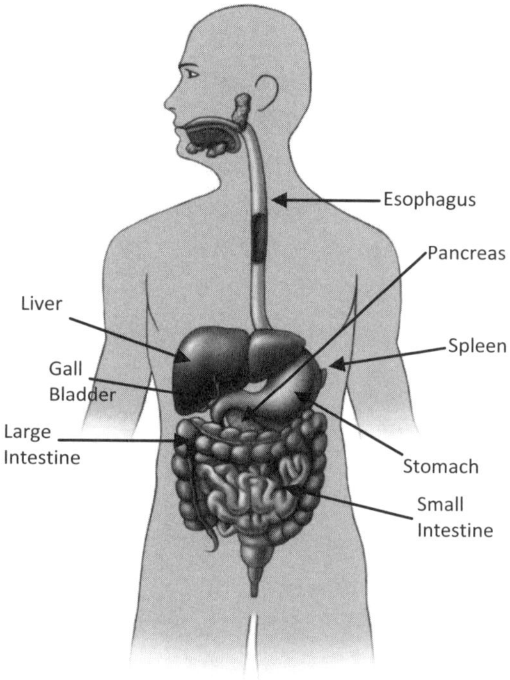

Blood Pressure Problems

High and low blood pressure may have several potential causes, however what follows are the basic mechanics. Blood pressure is obviously regulated by the Heart; it is also regulated by the Liver and the Kidney/Adrenal system.

High Blood Pressure

The Liver has 600 physiological functions, of which one is to help the body cope with life's emotional stresses. Another of the Liver's functions is to drive the blood and energy freely through the body in a relaxed fashion. In other words, if the Liver is functioning well, the blood vessels are relaxed and stable. In addition, the Liver "nourishes" Heart function (the Heart has an important role in high blood pressure; however, the Heart derives much of its function from the Liver).

An example follows: one experiences long-lasting emotional stress and eventually the Liver starts to break down, leading to decreased Heart function. The blood vessels begin to contract, over time becoming rigid. With the same volume of blood in now inelastic blood vessels, the pressure increases; hence, high blood pressure.

It is very common for a conventional Western Medical doctor to explain: "Stress in your life is causing high blood pressure," without fully understanding the exact sequence of events in the body that would cause one experiencing "stress" to have high blood pressure.

Low Blood Pressure

Generally, the successful treatment of low blood pressure involves building the affected organ systems' function until they are functioning normally as well as taking the following applicable sections into account[2].

Categories of blood pressure problems:

1. **High systolic** and **high diastolic** numbers with a **high pulse rate**, indicating "heat" and/or toxicity is trapped internally.

2. **Low systolic** and **low diastolic** numbers with a **slow pulse rate**, indicating the hot, invigorating aspect of the body is depleted. In such as case one must increase internal "heat" and increase circulation dramatically.

3. **High systolic** and **normal to high diastolic** numbers with a **slow pulse rate**, indicating blood circulation is stagnating and that "empty heat" exists. In such a case one must increase blood circulation dramatically and build the cool, moist, nourishing aspect of the body.

---

[2] Chang, Jimmy Wei-Yen and Brinkman, Marcus, *Pulsesynergy: A Pulse Diagnosis Manual*, 1995. 166p.

4. **Low systolic** and **low diastolic** numbers with a **rapid Heart rate**, indicating "empty heat" exists. In this case, one must build the cool, moist, nourishing aspect of the body.

Given that one of the Liver's 600 functions is to purify the bloodstream, reducing or eliminating the intake of toxic chemicals is very important as part of a larger strategy to resolve high blood pressure. Given that the Heart and Liver are likely involved at least to some degree, it is important to exercise gently (under the supervision of your doctor) for at least 30 minutes four times weekly, thus increasing circulation, soothing the Heart and Liver and stimulating increased circulation throughout the body, which allows the blood vessels to relax.

As you can see with this particular health problem, there is an underlying cause. The key to success in treating these problems lies in addressing the underlying issue described above to eliminate the problem over the long term. To speed Acupuncture and/or Chinese Herbal Medicine results, it is recommended one minimally reduce or eliminate the intake of caffeine, deep-fried foods, dairy, sugar, preservatives in food, chemicals in food and municipal tap water (which most often contains chlorine and fluoride, considered by many as dangerous chemicals).

Bursitis

Bursitis has many potential causes, however what follows are the basic mechanics. Bursitis involves inflammation of the bursa, which are sacs of fluid between tendons and bones in joints such as the knee, elbow or shoulder. The inflammation is often a result of repetitive motion or physical trauma.

Acupuncture promotes healing of the bursa by encouraging circulation into the area to drive out the inflammation. Eventually, the bursa will return to its normal state, eliminating the source of the pain.

As you can see with this particular health problem, there is an underlying cause. The key to success in treating these problems lies in addressing the underlying issue described above to eliminate the problem over the long term. To speed Acupuncture and/or Chinese Herbal Medicine results, it is recommended one minimally reduce or eliminate the intake of caffeine, deep-fried foods, dairy, sugar, preservatives in food, chemicals in food and municipal tap water (which most often contains chlorine and fluoride, considered by many as dangerous chemicals).

Cancer

Obviously cancer has many potential causes, however what follows are the basic mechanics at work. In Oriental Medicine over that last several thousand years, an understanding of fluids in the body has developed. Essentially food and fluids are ingested; those foods and fluids are supposed to be broken down and distributed throughout the body and used for multiple purposes. There is a scale regarding fluids in the body that have "gone awry" in the process of fluid metabolism and distribution. Below is what is called the "Tan-Yin Scale."

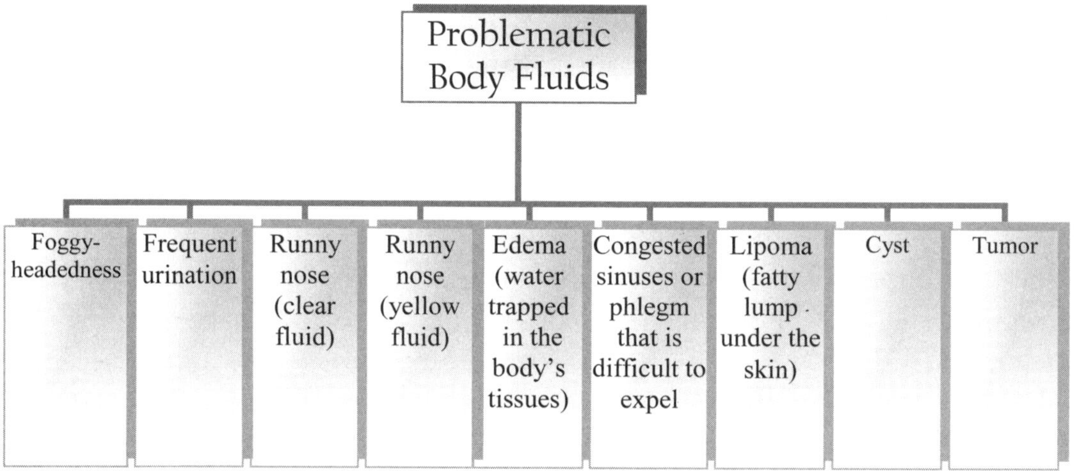

At the far left end of this spectrum would be a feeling of "foggy-headedness." Other more dense forms of fluids not being fully metabolized include edema, nasal discharge, cough with minimal phlegm, cough with a lot of phlegm, swollen ankles and sinus congestion.

Moving down to the scale on the right end of the spectrum, now you have someone who has an excess fatty tissue. Going down further down the scale to the right would be a lipoma (a fatty lump under the surface of the skin) or a cyst. Finally, there would be a benign or even malignant tumor, the densest example of fluids on this scale. Cancerous cells are basically fluids that are very inefficiently metabolized that become "moldy" over time as the body is loaded with toxicity and dangerous material.

As you can see with this particular health problem, there is an underlying cause. The key to success in treating these problems lies in addressing the underlying issue described above to eliminate the problem over the long term. To speed Acupuncture and/or Chinese Herbal Medicine results, it is recommended one minimally reduce or eliminate the intake of caffeine, deep-fried foods, dairy, sugar, preservatives in food, chemicals in food and municipal tap water (which most often contains chlorine and fluoride, considered by many as dangerous chemicals).

Carpal Tunnel Syndrome

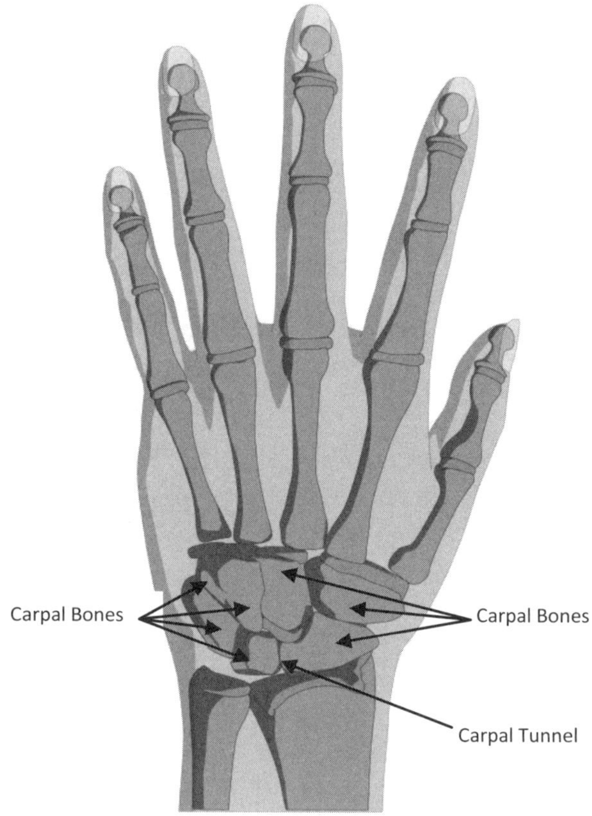

Carpal tunnel syndrome (the carpal tunnel is a passageway filled with ligaments, tendons, nerves, and bones at the base of the hand) may be caused by the following[3]:

1. A lack of the body's nourishing fluids, wherein they are not lubricating the wrist joint properly (likened to an inadequately lubricated door hinge), causing pain.

2. A thickening from irritated tendons.

---

[3] U.S. National Library of Medicine and National Institutes of Health, Carpal Tunnel Syndrome, http://www.nlm.nih.gov/medlineplus/carpaltunnelsyndrome.html (Accessed December, 2010).

3. Swelling of other tissues that cause the nerve to be compressed.

As you can see with this particular health problem, there is an underlying cause. The key to success in treating these problems lies in addressing the underlying issue described above to eliminate the problem over the long term. To speed Acupuncture and/or Chinese Herbal Medicine results, it is recommended one minimally reduce or eliminate the intake of caffeine, deep-fried foods, dairy, sugar, preservatives in food, chemicals in food and municipal tap water (which most often contains chlorine and fluoride, considered by many as dangerous chemicals).

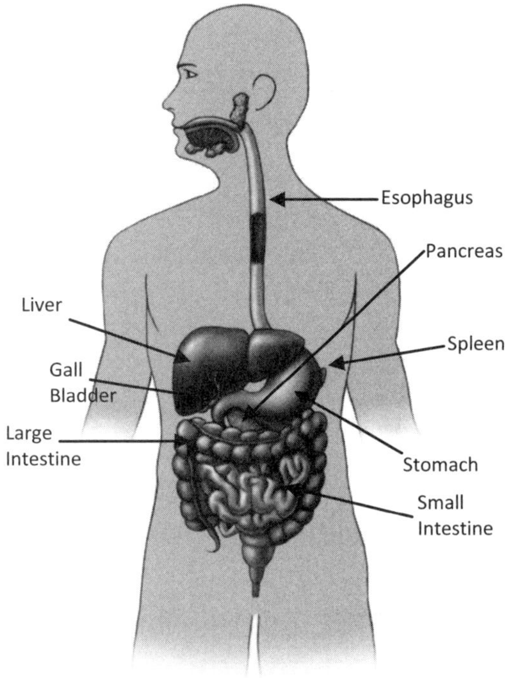

Cholesterol Problems

Cholesterol imbalances have many potential causes, however what follows are the basic mechanics.

The Liver has 600 physiological functions, of which one is helping the body to metabolize and use fats in the food one consumes. The Spleen/Pancreatic system has many functions, one of which is to help the body to metabolize food and fluids that you consume, making those things useable by the body. A loss of Liver and/or Spleen/Pancreatic function may cause cholesterol abnormalities.

Given that one of the Liver's 600 functions is to purify the bloodstream, reducing or eliminating the intake of toxic chemicals is very important as part of a larger strategy to treat and/ or prevent cholesterol imbalances. It is also important to exercise vigorously (to a point of perspiration) for at least 30 minutes four times weekly, thus increasing Liver circulation, soothing the Liver and stimulating increased circulation throughout the body, which allows the body to detoxify at least to a small degree.

As you can see with this particular health problem, there is an underlying cause. The key to success in treating these problems lies in addressing the underlying issue described above to eliminate the problem over the long term. To speed Acupuncture and/or Chinese Herbal Medicine results, it is recommended one minimally reduce or eliminate the intake of caffeine, deep-fried foods, dairy, sugar, preservatives in food, chemicals in food and municipal tap water (which most often contains chlorine and fluoride, considered by many as dangerous chemicals).

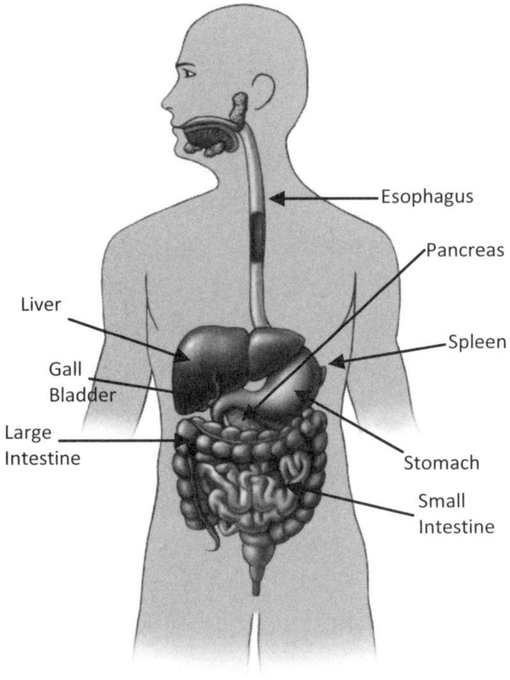

Constipation

Constipation has many potential causes, however what follows are some of the basic mechanics.

1. In many cases there may be excess "heat" in the body, causing fluids to evaporate, leading to dense, dry stool that moves with difficulty.

2. It may also be caused by such Large Intestine and Small Intestine weakness that they cannot properly move the stool through.

3. It is also possible that when not adapting to stress, the Liver may "overact" on the intestinal tract, causing constriction in the intestine and a lack of peristalsis (successive waves of contractions in the intestine walls that propel stool through and eventually out of the body).

4. Yet another possible cause is a Heart and Small Intestine imbalance, which may be oftentimes triggered by mental and emotional stress.

Constipation is a condition to be resolved as quickly as possible; if stool remains in the intestinal tract for longer than 18 hours, toxins from the stool will move through the intestine wall into the bloodstream, polluting the entire body.

As you can see with this particular health problem, there is an underlying cause. The key to success in treating these problems lies in addressing the underlying issue described above to eliminate the problem over the long term. To speed Acupuncture and/or Chinese Herbal Medicine results, it is recommended one minimally reduce or eliminate the intake of caffeine, deep-fried foods, dairy, sugar, preservatives in food, chemicals in food and municipal tap water (which most often contains chlorine and fluoride, considered by many as dangerous chemicals).

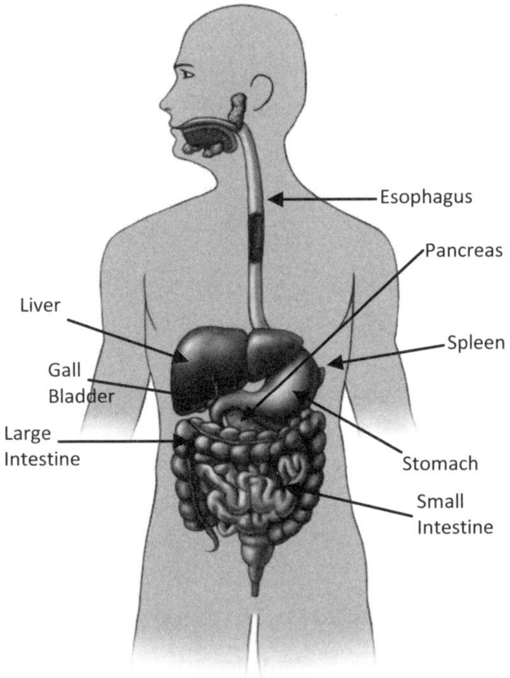

Depression

Depression has many potential causes, however what follows are the basic mechanics. Thousands of years ago, physicians in China began to explore the nature of human emotion and discovered a direct link between emotion and the organ system. Having helped many people resolve emotional imbalances over the years, we've found the following to be accurate from the point of view of the physical body (obviously many factors exist in life that may trigger bodily malfunction which, in turn, could then trigger an emotional response). What is described below is the relationship between the emotions and physical body.

The Liver has 600 physiological functions, one of which is to help the body adapt to the mental and emotional stresses of life. In other words, if one's Liver is functioning at a high level, stress entering one's life has no physical effect; however, if one's Liver isn't functioning well, stress can have a negative effect on the body.

Liver malfunction can cause a person to experience excessive or inappropriate anger, irritability, frustration, impatience, and/or depression. For example, a person with multiple emotional stresses over many years may experience suppressed Liver function. Then, the loss of a loved one could cause Liver function to drop dramatically, and the person could then begin to experience depression. On the other hand, a well-functioning Liver will cause one to be emotionally even and generally happy.

Depression can be caused by a breakdown in Liver function, not simply an imbalance in brain chemistry (the typical Western Medical view of this particular condition). Ironically, addressing only the brain chemistry with medication often leads to further difficulty resolving the problem as shown here: if one takes a medication for depression (which may be caused by a Liver imbalance) and that medication reduces Liver function (the Liver, in its capacity as a blood purifier, will attempt to eliminate the chemical from the body), it makes it more difficult to treat the depression. This explains why a person may take a medication their entire life.....and the depression never fully resolves!

Given that one of the Liver's 600 functions is to purify the bloodstream, reducing or eliminating the intake of toxic chemicals is very important as part of a larger strategy to resolve depression. It is also important to exercise vigorously (to a point of perspiration) for at least 30 minutes four times weekly, thus increasing Liver circulation, soothing the Liver and stimulating increased circulation throughout the body, which allows the body to detoxify at least to a small degree.

As you can see with this particular health problem, there is an underlying cause. The key to success in treating these problems lies in addressing the underlying issue described above to eliminate the problem over the long term. To speed Acupuncture and/or Chinese Herbal Medicine results, it is recommended one minimally reduce or eliminate the intake of caffeine, deep-fried foods, dairy, sugar, preservatives in food, chemicals in food and municipal tap water (which most often contains chlorine and fluoride, considered by many as dangerous chemicals).

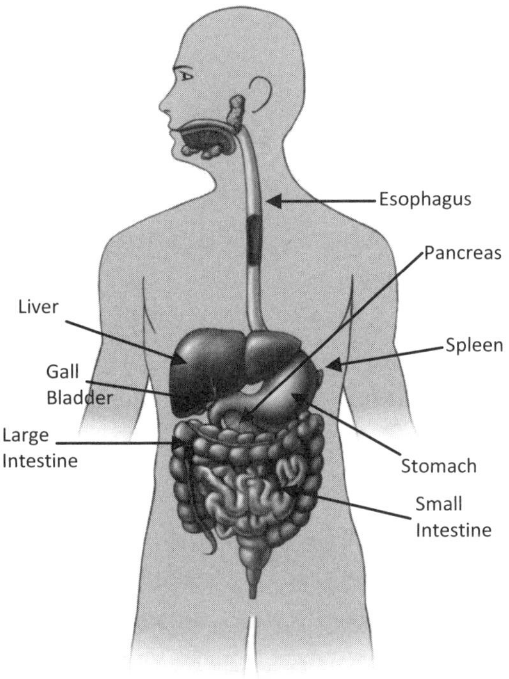

Diabetes

Diabetes obviously has many potential causes, however what follows are the basic mechanics.

Conventional Western Medicine recognizes two forms of diabetes: Type I diabetes (called "insulin-dependent" or "juvenile" diabetes) involves impaired insulin production by the Spleen/Pancreatic system, typically occurring before the age of 25. Type II (referred to as "non-insulin-dependent" or "adult-onset" diabetes) involves diminished tissue sensitivity to insulin and possibly may also involve impaired Spleen/Pancreatic function and may be worsened by obesity.

Essentially, the Spleen/Pancreatic system manufactures insulin and releases it into the blood stream to pull glucose (sugar) into the cell, giving one energy. If the Spleen/Pancreatic system's function declines, it cannot produce the insulin necessary to handle glucose in the blood stream, which causes a variety of diabetic symptoms.

Spleen/Pancreatic system function responds favorably to Oriental Medical care in many cases, thus normalizing insulin and glucose levels in Type I and Type II diabetes.

As you can see with this particular health problem, there is an underlying cause. The key to success in treating these problems lies in addressing the underlying issue described above to eliminate the problem over the long term. To speed Acupuncture and/or Chinese Herbal Medicine results, it is recommended one minimally reduce or eliminate the intake of caffeine, deep-fried foods, dairy, sugar, simple carbohydrates, preservatives in food, chemicals in food and municipal tap water (which most often contains chlorine and fluoride, considered by many as dangerous chemicals).

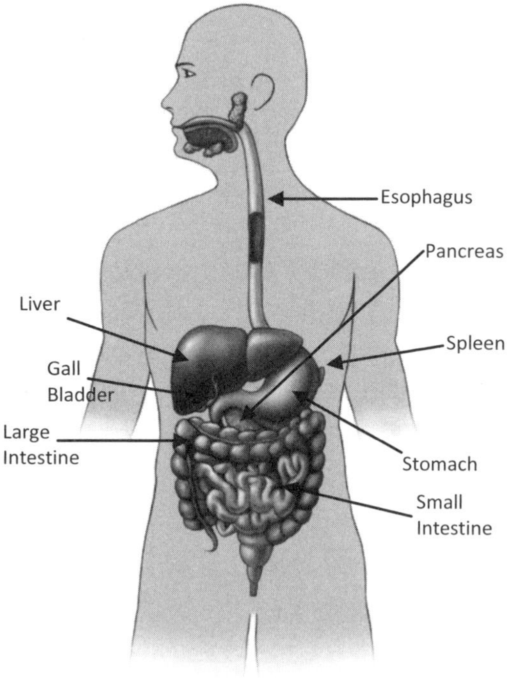

Digestive Problems (General)

Digestive problems take many forms and have many potential causes, however what follows are the basic mechanics. The Stomach receives the food and fluids one consumes via the esophagus and the Spleen/Pancreatic system (which also manufactures insulin, produces certain immune system cells) breaks down that food and fluid into usable nutrients that are sent to the intestines where they travel into the bloodstream through the intestine wall. The Liver produces bile which the Gall Bladder releases into the intestines to dissolve fats that you consume. The Small Intestine separates usable parts of food and fluids from the unusable, distributes the usable components throughout the body and eliminates the unusable components. Finally, the Large Intestine eliminates solid waste from the body.

Given that one of the Liver's 600 functions is to purify the bloodstream, reducing or eliminating the intake of toxic chemicals is very important as part of a larger strategy to resolve digestive problems. It is also important to exercise vigorously (to a point of perspiration) for at least 30 minutes four times weekly, thus increasing Liver circulation, soothing the Liver and stimulating increased circulation throughout the body, which allows the body to detoxify at least to a small degree.

As you can see with this particular health problem, there is an underlying cause. The key to success in treating these problems lies in addressing the underlying issue described above to eliminate the problem over the long term. To speed Acupuncture and/or Chinese Herbal Medicine results, it is recommended one minimally reduce or eliminate the intake of caffeine, deep-fried foods, dairy, sugar, preservatives in food, chemicals in food and municipal tap water (which most often contains chlorine and fluoride, considered by many as dangerous chemicals).

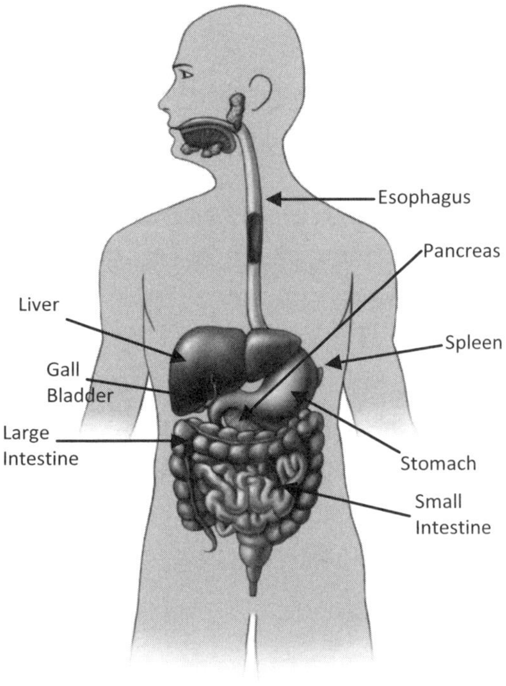

Diarrhea

Chronic diarrhea has many potential causes, however what follows are the basic mechanics. Diarrhea is most often caused by too many fluids in the stool; that fluid may derive from many sources. In many cases the "digestive fire" is weak and unable to evaporate fluids from the stool, and the excess water in the stool leads to diarrhea.

There are five basic types of diarrhea:

1. Diarrhea caused by the Stomach is often yellowish with undigested material.

2. Diarrhea caused by the Spleen/Pancreatic system may cause watery stool, abdominal swelling and/or possible vomiting after eating. The Kidney/Adrenal system may also be involved in such cases.

3. Diarrhea caused by the Large Intestine will often involve acute abdominal swelling after meals with potentially white appearing stools. There may be rumbling and/or a "slicing" type of pain accompanying bowel movements.

4. Diarrhea caused by the Small Intestine may present with blood in the stool and/or the urine and may be accompanied by pain in the lower abdomen.

5. Dysentery causes a desire to have a bowel movement without being able to evacuate the bowels. There also may be sensations of lower digestive pain and a feeling of the lower digestive system "falling."

As you can see with this particular health problem, there is an underlying cause. The key to success in treating these problems lies in addressing the underlying issue described above to eliminate the problem over the long term. To speed Acupuncture and/or Chinese Herbal Medicine results, it is recommended one minimally reduce or eliminate the intake of caffeine, deep-fried foods, dairy, sugar, preservatives in food, chemicals in food and municipal tap water (which most often contains chlorine and fluoride, considered by many as dangerous chemicals).

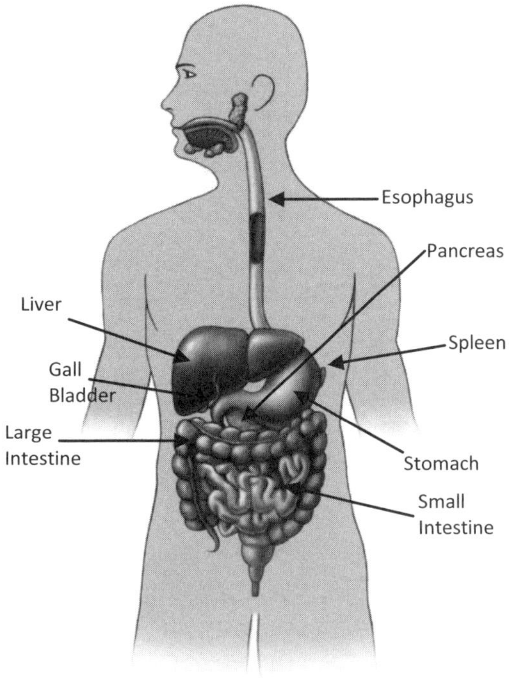

Diverticulitis

Diverticulitis (a condition involving inflamed abnormal sacs that protrude outward from the intestines) is most often caused by the accumulation of an extraordinary amount of toxins and/or chemicals from foods and fluids that people eat and drink. These toxins build up in the intestines and the body isolates the material in small pockets that become inflamed and agitated.

As you can see with this particular health problem, there is an underlying cause. The key to success in treating these problems lies in addressing the underlying issue described above to eliminate the problem over the long term. To speed Acupuncture and/or Chinese Herbal Medicine results, it is recommended one minimally reduce or eliminate the intake of caffeine, deep-fried foods, dairy, sugar, preservatives in food, chemicals in food and municipal tap water (which most often contains chlorine and fluoride, considered by many as dangerous chemicals).

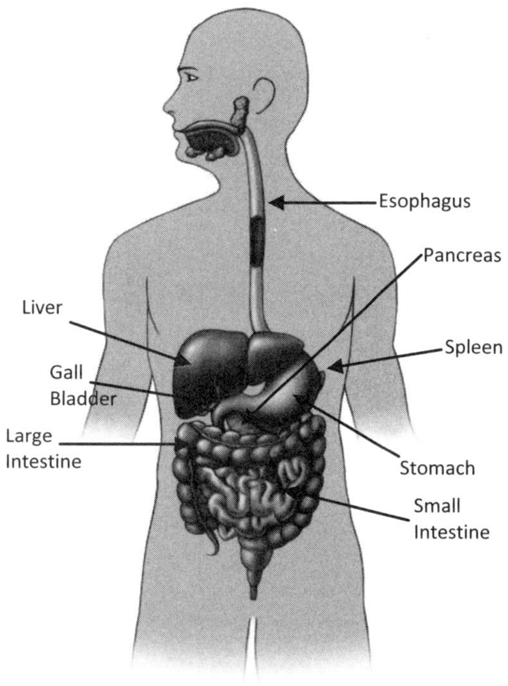

Dizziness and Vertigo

Dizziness and vertigo have many potential causes, however what follows are the two most likely possible causes.

1. A lack of volume of blood in the body (therefore a lack of oxygen in the brain) may lead to dizziness and/or vertigo. For example, if one experiences dizziness upon standing from a sitting position, it may indicate the body does not possess the volume of blood necessary to push adequate blood quickly enough into the brain to compensate for the body movement.

2. The Liver has 600 physiological functions, one of which is to help the body adapt to the mental and emotional stresses of life. In other words, if one's Liver is functioning at a high level, stress entering one's life has no physical effect; however, if one's Liver isn't functioning well, stress can have a negative effect on the body. If the Liver has lost function, it may

break down under the emotional stresses and traumas of life and excess circulation from the Liver may ascend to the head, causing dizziness and/or vertigo.

As you can see with this particular health problem, there is an underlying cause. The key to success in treating these problems lies in addressing the underlying issue described above to eliminate the problem over the long term. To speed Acupuncture and/or Chinese Herbal Medicine results, it is recommended one minimally reduce or eliminate the intake of caffeine, deep-fried foods, dairy, sugar, preservatives in food, chemicals in food and municipal tap water (which most often contains chlorine and fluoride, considered by many as dangerous chemicals).

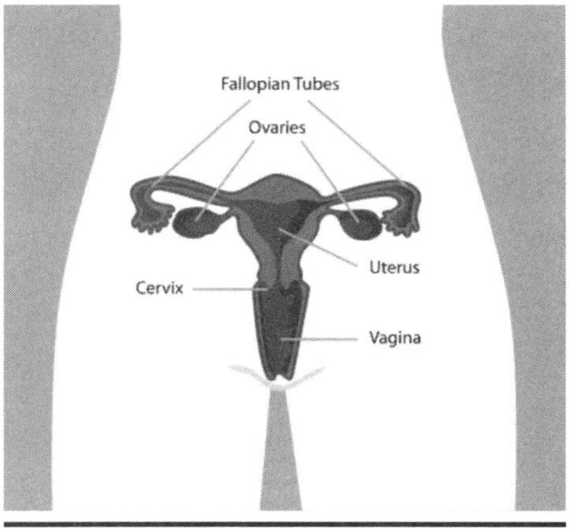

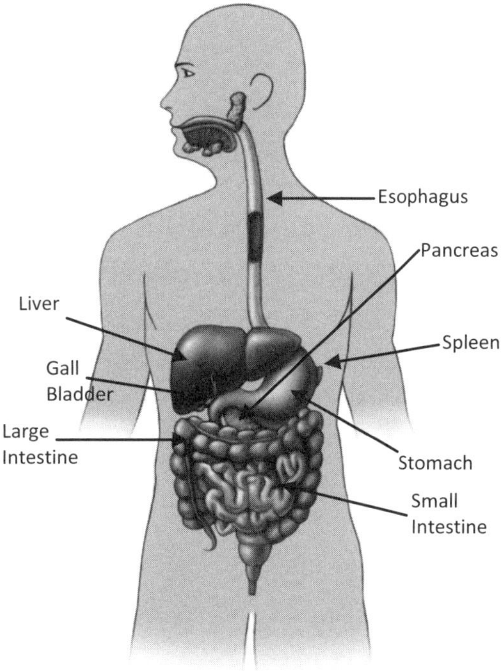

Endometriosis

Endometriosis has many potential causes, however what follows are the basic mechanics.

The Liver has 600 physiological functions, one being to encourage the free flow of blood and energy everywhere in the body. Endometriosis is a result of the inside lining of the uterus moving into the abdominal cavity with a simultaneous breakdown in Liver function, causing blood to coagulate into a web-like matrix of material in the abdominal cavity.

Another of the Liver's functions is to purify the bloodstream, therefore, reducing or eliminating the intake of toxic chemicals is very important as part of a larger strategy to resolve Endometriosis. It is also important to exercise vigorously (to a point of perspiration) for at least 30 minutes four times weekly, thus increasing Liver circulation, soothing the Liver and stimulating increased circulation throughout the body, which allows the body to detoxify at least to a small degree.

As you can see with this particular health problem, there is an underlying cause. The key to success in treating these problems lies in addressing the underlying issue described above to eliminate the problem over the long term. To speed Acupuncture and/or Chinese Herbal Medicine results, it is recommended one minimally reduce or eliminate the intake of caffeine, deep-fried foods, dairy, sugar, preservatives in food, chemicals in food and municipal tap water (which most often contains chlorine and fluoride, considered by many as dangerous chemicals).

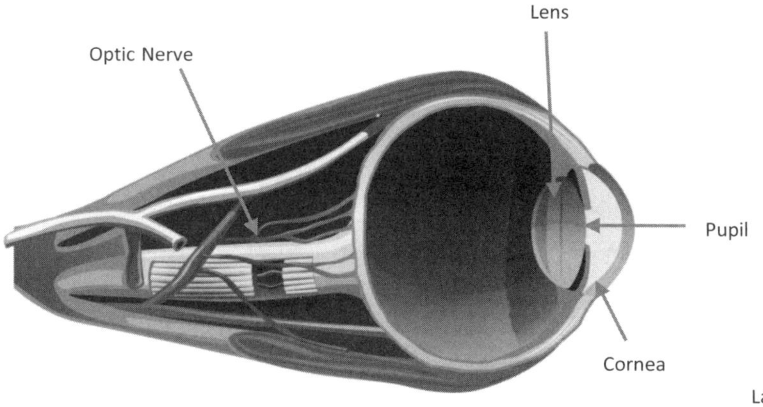

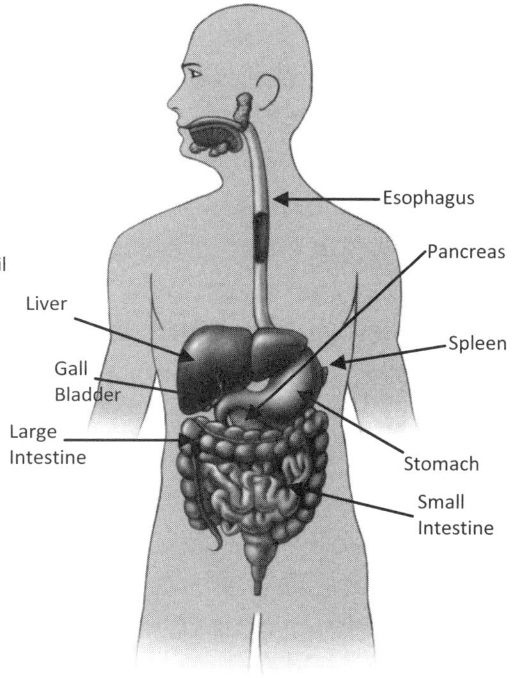

Eye Problems: Dry Eyes, Itchy Eyes, Gritty Eyes, Blurry Vision, Floaters, Double Vision, Visual Disturbances, Ocular Migraines, Etc.

Eye problems and their causes are varied, however what follows are the basic mechanics. An incident (for example, a traumatic injury) can damage the eye, leading to such symptoms. On the other hand, the Liver--which "nourishes" and "opens" to the eyes as two of its 600 physiological functions--can cause a wide variety of eye problems.

In the case of injury, Acupuncture speeds healing of the tissues locally to reinstate normal eye function. In the case of Liver malfunction causing the eye problems, Acupuncture reinstates normal Liver function to resolve the eye issue.

Another of the Liver's functions is to purify the bloodstream, therefore, reducing or eliminating the intake of toxic chemicals is very important as part of a larger strategy to resolve eye problems. It is also important to exercise vigorously (to a point of perspiration) for at least 30 minutes four times weekly, thus increasing Liver circulation, soothing the Liver and stimulating increased circulation throughout the body, which allows the body to detoxify at least to a small degree.

As you can see with this particular health problem, there is an underlying cause. The key to success in treating these problems lies in addressing the underlying issue described above to eliminate the problem over the long term. To speed Acupuncture and/or Chinese Herbal Medicine results, it is recommended one minimally reduce or eliminate the intake of caffeine, deep-fried foods, dairy, sugar, preservatives in food, chemicals in food and municipal tap water (which most often contains chlorine and fluoride, considered by many as dangerous chemicals).

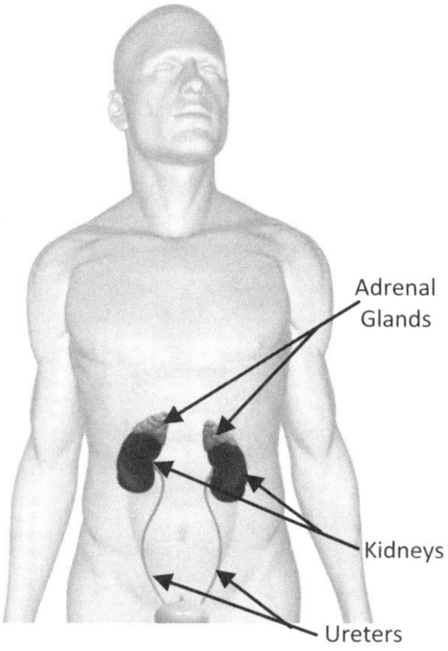

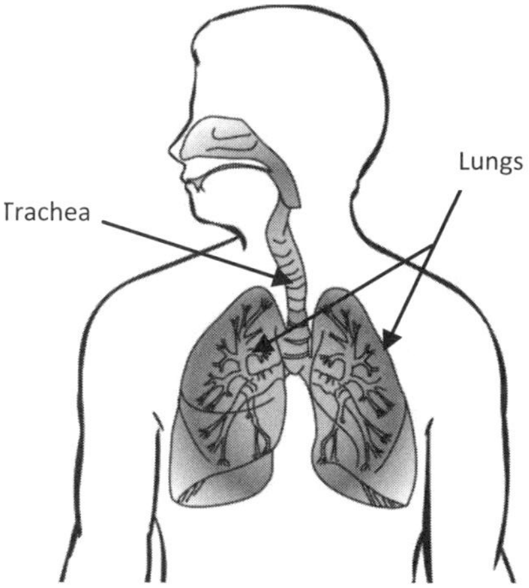

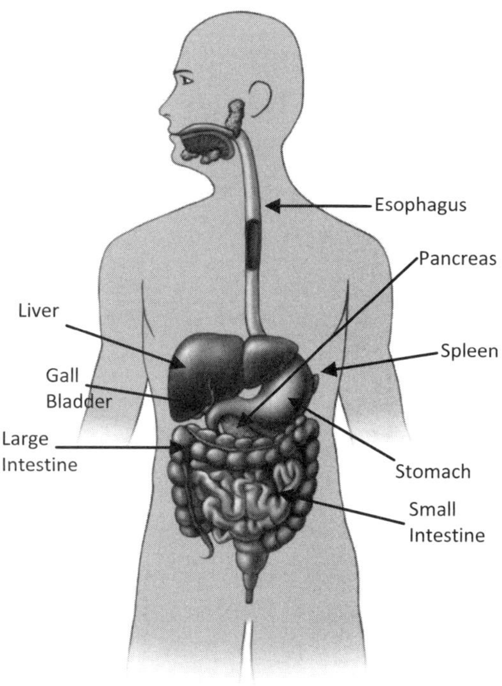

Fatigue

Fatigue has many potential causes, however what follows are the basic mechanics. Several organs produce and distribute energy throughout the body.

1. The Stomach, Spleen/Pancreatic system are responsible for a certain amount of energy production, which begins as food is broken down into nutrients in the Stomach, in part due to the actions of the Spleen/Pancreatic system. Those nutrients are then sent into the intestines, pass through the intestine wall into the blood stream and travel throughout the body, stimulating processes that give energy. Regardless of how well one eats, lack of Stomach and/or Spleen/Pancreatic system function will often lead to fatigue.

2. The Lungs may be involved with fatigue; one of the Lungs' functions is to bring oxygen into the body, which then travels in the bloodstream to the brain giving energy. Thus, a lack of Lung function may cause fatigue.

3. The Kidney/Adrenal system (which produces and releases adrenaline) may be depleted by long-term inadequate sleep, excessive mental stress and/or excessive physical stress, possibly leading to fatigue.

4. The Heart (which is responsible for driving oxygen-laden blood throughout the body) may malfunction, leading to reduced oxygen in the brain, thus causing fatigue.

As you can see with this particular health problem, there is an underlying cause. The key to success in treating these problems lies in addressing the underlying issue described above to eliminate the problem over the long term. To speed Acupuncture and/or Chinese Herbal Medicine results, it is recommended that one increase protein in ratio to carbohydrates at every meal and minimally reduce or eliminate the intake of caffeine, deep-fried foods, dairy, sugar, preservatives in food, chemicals in food and municipal tap water (which most often contains chlorine and fluoride, considered by many as dangerous chemicals).

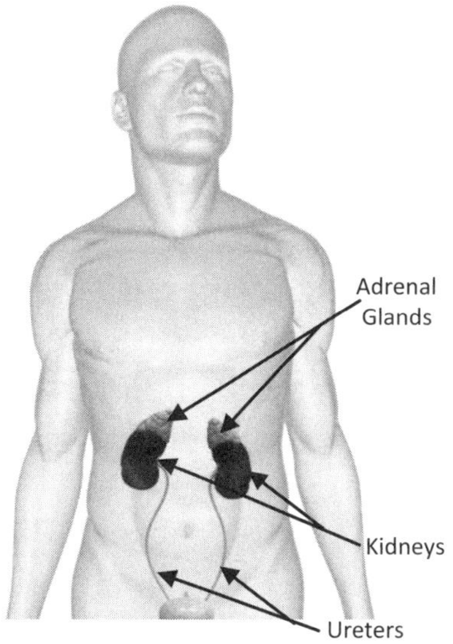

Fibromyalgia

Fibromyalgia has many potential causes, however what follows are the basic mechanics. "Fibro" comes from *fiber* or *fibrous-* the body's soft tissues under the skin, especially around the joints, including tendons. "My" comes from *myo-* meaning muscles. "Alg" comes from *algos-* meaning pain. "Ia" means "state of/condition." This is a conventional Western Medicine diagnosis wherein a patient experiences 11 of 18 tender/painful points (acupuncture points, actually), fatigue, depression and other related symptoms.

Normally, blood and energy flow freely throughout the body. Sharp and/or fixed pain indicates improper blood circulation; dull and/or generalized pain indicates improper energy circulation; shooting and/or "electric" pain indicates nervous system problems.

In many cases, the *underlying* cause of the pain is a Kidney/Adrenal system imbalance. The Kidney/Adrenal system is the root of the "yin" and the "yang" of the body. The yin is the cool, moist and nourishing aspect of the body (for example the amniotic fluid around the baby in the womb) whereas yang is very moving and invigorating (an example of yang gone "awry" is a woman having a hot flash). If there is a lack of yang, it may not be able to *drive* the blood and energy *throughout* the entire body.

As you can see with this particular health problem, there is an underlying cause. The key to success in treating these problems lies in addressing the underlying issue described above to eliminate the problem over the long term. To speed Acupuncture and/or Chinese Herbal Medicine results, it is recommended one minimally reduce or eliminate the intake of caffeine, deep-fried foods, dairy, sugar, preservatives in food, chemicals in food and municipal tap water (which most often contains chlorine and fluoride, considered by many as dangerous chemicals).

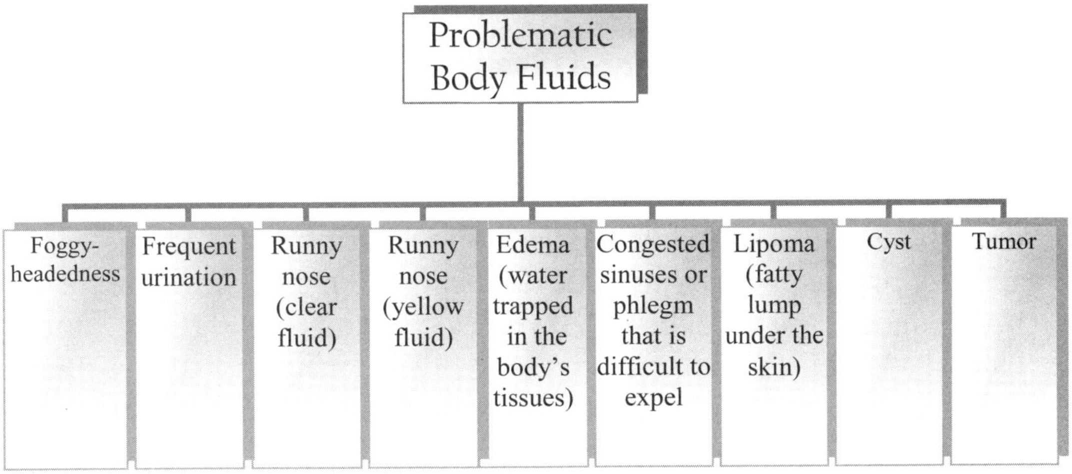

Fluid Metabolism and Distribution Problems

In Oriental Medicine there exists a scale (see above) that illustrates various forms of fluids in the body may take when they are not fully metabolized or distributed appropriately, which is often caused by Kidney/Adrenal system malfunction, Spleen/Pancreatic system malfunction, or Lung malfunction.

At one end of this scale, one experiences the most subtle, invisible form of fluids: a feeling of "foggy-headedness" (a feeling as if one has cotton in one's head), perhaps experienced on a rainy day. Further to the right on the scale, one may experience frequent urination. A bit further to the right on the scale, one experiences a runny nose with clear fluid. Further to the right one experiences nasal discharge with thick, yellow fluids. A little further to the right, one experience symptoms such as edema: swollen ankles, abdominal bloating, and/or inflamed sinuses with fluids underneath the surface of the mucus membranes. Even further to the right, one may experience a small lipoma (a soft, round or oval deposit of fatty material that grows under the skin). Further to the right still, one may experience a cyst; and finally, at the extreme right end of the scale would be a tumor that is fixed in location, dense, and potentially dangerous.

As you can see with this particular health problem, there is an underlying cause. The key to success in treating these problems lies in addressing the underlying issue described above to eliminate the problem over the long term. To speed Acupuncture and/or Chinese Herbal Medicine results, it is recommended one minimally reduce or eliminate the intake of caffeine, deep-fried foods, dairy, sugar, preservatives in food, excessive raw vegetables and other foods, chemicals in food and municipal tap water (which most often contains chlorine and fluoride, considered by many as dangerous chemicals).

Foot/Ankle Problems

There are many potential causes of foot pain, however what follows are four basic possibilities. Additionally, it is important to note that the Kidney/Adrenal system governs the function of the feet.

1. Nerve damage in the foot may cause a person to experience strange sensations, such as a feeling of "walking on pebbles" or "bubble wrap."

2. A lack of blood volume in the foot may cause a sensation of numbness.

3. Decreased energy circulation in the foot may cause dull pain.

4. Severe blood stagnation and/or scar tissue (see the section "Pain Due to Scar Tissue") in the foot may cause sharp pain.

Any or all of the above may be involved when one experiences foot pain.

As you can see with this particular health problem, there is an underlying cause. The key to success in treating these problems lies in addressing the underlying issue described above to eliminate the problem over the long term. To speed Acupuncture and/or Chinese Herbal Medicine results, it is recommended one minimally reduce or eliminate the intake of caffeine, deep-fried foods, dairy, sugar, preservatives in food, excessive raw vegetables and other foods, chemicals in food and municipal tap water (which most often contains chlorine and fluoride, considered by many as dangerous chemicals).

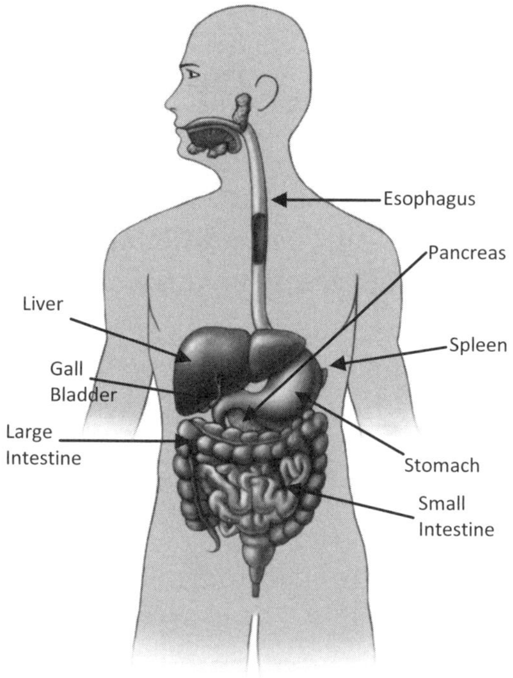

Frustration

Excessive and/or inappropriate frustration has many potential causes, however what follows are the basic mechanics. Thousands of years ago, physicians in China began to explore the nature of human emotion and discovered a direct link between emotion and the organ system. Having helped many people resolve emotional imbalances over the years, we've found the following to be accurate from the point of view of the physical body (obviously many factors exist in life that may trigger bodily malfunction which, in turn, could then trigger an emotional response). What is described below is the relationship between the emotions and physical body.

The Liver has 600 physiological functions, one of which is to help the body adapt to the mental and emotional stresses of life. In other words, if one's Liver is functioning at a high level, stress entering one's life has no physical effect; however, if one's Liver isn't functioning well, stress can have a negative effect on the body.

Liver malfunction can cause a person to experience excessive or inappropriate anger, irritability, frustration, impatience, and/or depression. For example, a person with multiple emotional stresses over many years may experience suppressed Liver function. Then, the loss of a loved one could cause Liver function to drop dramatically, and the person could then begin to experience inappropriate and/or excessive frustration. On the other hand, a well-functioning Liver will cause one to be emotionally even and generally happy.

Excessive or inappropriate frustration can be caused by a breakdown in Liver function, not simply an imbalance in brain chemistry (the typical Western Medical view of this particular condition). Ironically, addressing only the brain chemistry with medication often leads to further difficulty resolving the problem as shown here: if one takes a medication for excessive frustration (which may be caused by a Liver imbalance) and that medication reduces Liver function (the Liver, in its capacity as a blood purifier, will attempt to eliminate the chemical from the body), it makes it more difficult to treat the frustration. This explains why a person may take a medication their entire life.....and the frustration never fully resolves!

Given that one of the Liver's 600 functions is to purify the bloodstream, reducing or eliminating the intake of toxic chemicals is very important as part of a larger strategy to resolve frustration. It is also important to exercise vigorously (to a point of perspiration) for at least 30 minutes four times weekly, thus increasing Liver circulation, soothing the Liver and stimulating increased circulation throughout the body, which allows the body to detoxify at least to a small degree.

As you can see with this particular health problem, there is an underlying cause. The key to success in treating these problems lies in addressing the underlying issue described above to eliminate the problem over the long term. To speed Acupuncture and/or Chinese Herbal Medicine results, it is recommended one minimally reduce or eliminate the intake of caffeine, deep-fried foods, dairy, sugar,

preservatives in food, chemicals in food and municipal tap water (which most often contains chlorine and fluoride, considered by many as dangerous chemicals).

Hair loss

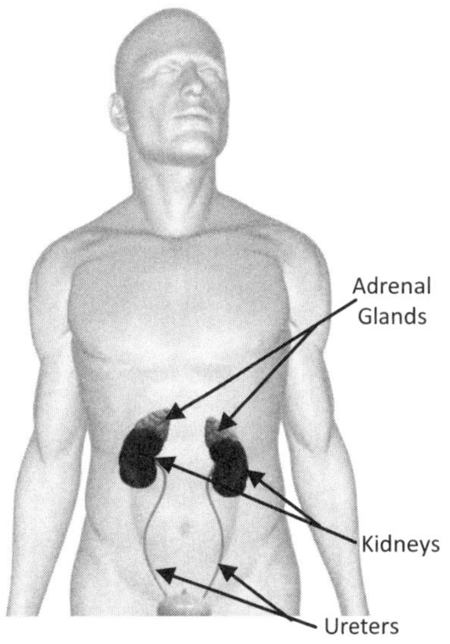

Hair loss has many potential causes, however what follows are the basic mechanics.

1. The Kidney/Adrenal system overall governs the production of hair; thus, a lack of Kidney/Adrenal function may lead to hair loss.

2. Adequate blood volume yields appropriate bloodstream nutrient content which nourishes the follicles (small glands in the scalp) which produce hair. Inadequate blood volume may lead to hair loss.

3. In some cases, toxins in the blood stream may travel to the follicle and destroy hair production.

As you can see with this particular health problem, there is an underlying cause. The key to success in treating these problems lies in addressing the underlying issue described above to eliminate the problem over the long term. To speed Acupuncture and/or Chinese Herbal Medicine results, it is recommended one minimally reduce or eliminate the intake of caffeine, deep-fried foods, dairy, sugar,

preservatives in food, chemicals in food and municipal tap water (which most often contains chlorine and fluoride, considered by many as dangerous chemicals).

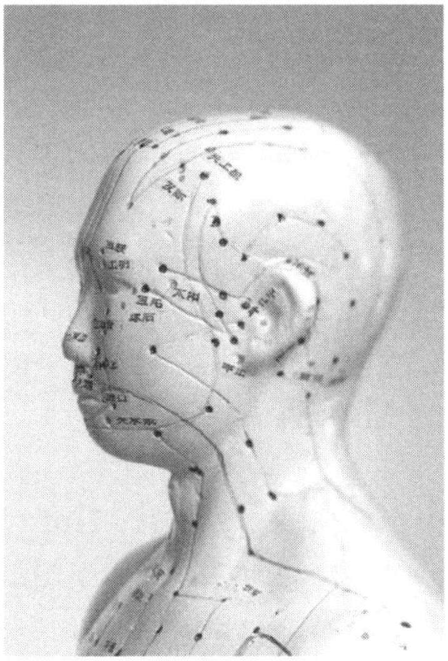

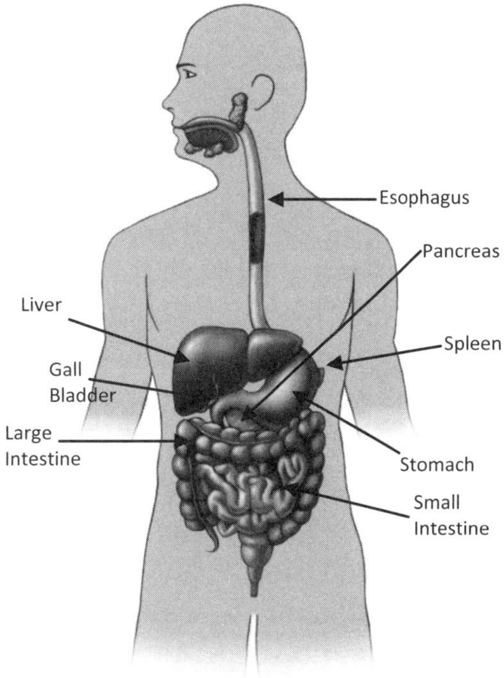

Headaches

Headaches have many potential causes, however what follows are the basic mechanics. Poor Liver and/or Gall Bladder function cause a significant number of headaches, as explained below.

The following illustrates the close relationship between the Liver and Gall Bladder as it relates to headaches: one of the Liver's 600 functions is to produce bile that is passed to the Gall Bladder and released into the intestine to "emulsify" (changing very large fat globules from food into much smaller fat droplets that can pass through the intestine wall and travel throughout the body in the bloodstream) fats upon consumption. The Liver also helps the body cope with life's emotional stresses and the Liver drives the blood and energy freely through the body in a relaxed fashion. In other words, if the Liver is functioning well, the blood vessels are relaxed and stable, whereas a loss of Liver function may lead to an inability to adapt to stress, resulting in blood vessel constriction, and finally Gall Bladder constriction, which may cause a referral of pain into the head, neck, and/or shoulders (see Gall Bladder connections to the head in the image above).

Headaches accompanied by eye and/or vision problems often indicate Liver involvement, as the Liver governs the functions of the eyes.

Digestive problems such as nausea that often accompany headaches may be caused by the Liver "overacting" on the digestive organs which, as you can see from the diagram above, are in very close proximity.

Given that another of the Liver's 600 functions is to purify the bloodstream, reducing or eliminating the intake of toxic chemicals is very important as part of a larger strategy to resolve headaches. It is also important to exercise vigorously (to a point of perspiration) for at least 30 minutes four times weekly, thus increasing Liver circulation, soothing the Liver and stimulating increased circulation throughout the body, which allows the body to detoxify at least to a small degree.

As you can see with this particular health problem, there is an underlying cause. The key to success in treating these problems lies in addressing the underlying issue described above to eliminate the problem over the long term. To speed Acupuncture and/or Chinese Herbal Medicine results, it is recommended one minimally reduce or eliminate the intake of caffeine, deep-fried foods, dairy, sugar, preservatives in food, chemicals in food and municipal tap water (which most often contains chlorine and fluoride, considered by many as dangerous chemicals).

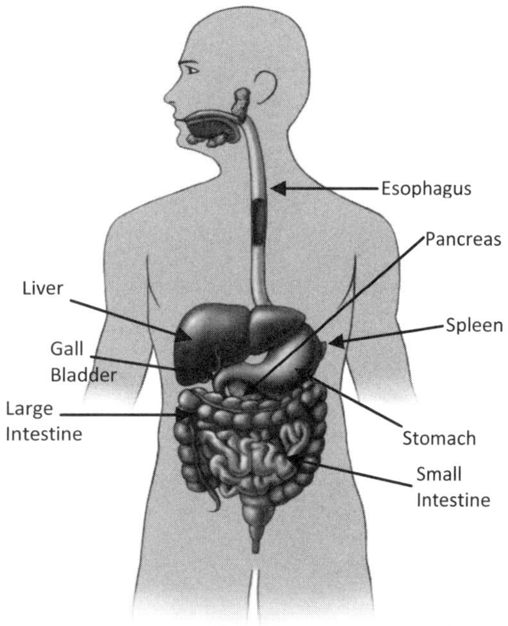

Hemorrhoids

Hemorrhoids have many potential causes, however what follows are the basic mechanics. The Spleen/Pancreatic system governs the function and structure of the blood vessels and is also in charge of "suspending the body's tissues in place" (such as blood vessels). Spleen/Pancreatic system malfunction may cause the veins to "sink" (prolapse) causing itchy, swollen and/or painful sensations in the lower rectum or anus. Obviously constipation may be a complicating factor, involving either the Large Intestine or Small Intestine.

As you can see with this particular health problem, there is an underlying cause. The key to success in treating these problems lies in addressing the underlying issue described above to eliminate the problem over the long term. To speed Acupuncture and/or Chinese Herbal Medicine results, it is recommended one minimally reduce or eliminate the intake of caffeine, deep-fried foods, dairy, sugar, preservatives in food, chemicals in food and municipal tap water (which most often contains chlorine and fluoride, considered by many as dangerous chemicals).

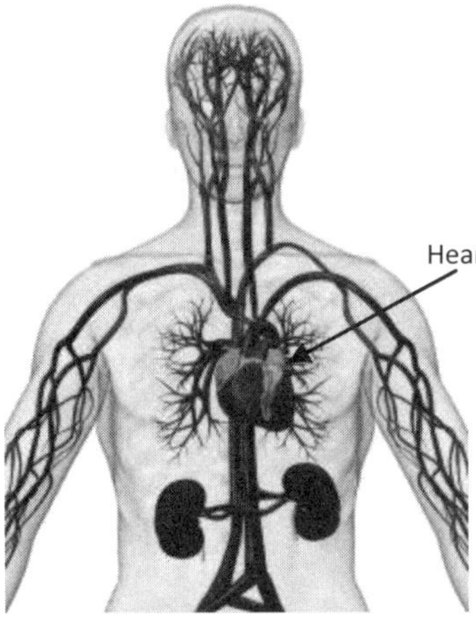

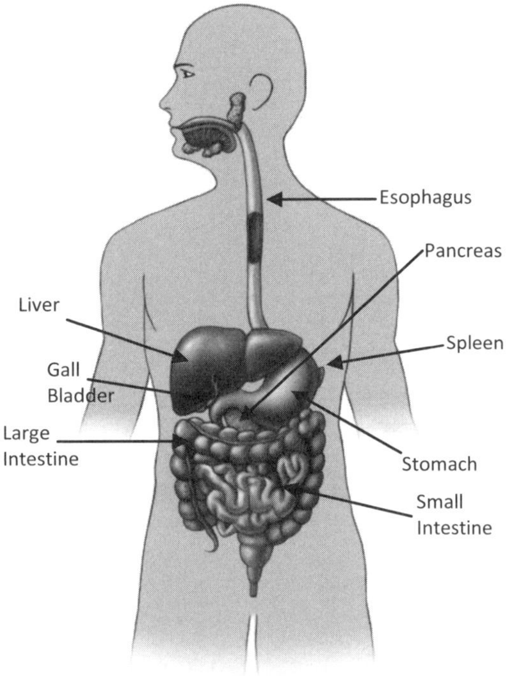

High Blood Pressure

High blood pressure has many potential causes, however what follows are the basic mechanics. Blood pressure is obviously regulated by the Heart, but also the Liver, and, to a certain degree, the Kidney/Adrenal system.

It is very common for a conventional Western Medical doctor to explain: "Stress in your life is causing high blood pressure," without fully understanding the exact sequence of events in the body that would cause one experiencing "stress" to have high blood pressure.

There exist four categories of blood pressure problems[4].

1. **High systolic** and **high diastolic** numbers with a **high pulse rate**, indicating "heat" and/or toxicity is trapped internally.

---

[4] Chang, Jimmy Wei-Yen and Brinkman, Marcus, *Pulsesynergy: A Pulse Diagnosis Manual*, 1995. 166p.

2. **Low systolic** and **low diastolic** numbers with a **slow pulse rate**, indicating the hot, invigorating aspect of the body is depleted. In such as case one must increase internal "heat" and increase circulation dramatically.

3. **High systolic** and **normal to high diastolic** numbers with a **slow pulse rate**, indicating blood circulation is stagnating and that "empty heat" exists. In such a case one must increase blood circulation dramatically and build the cool, moist, nourishing aspect of the body.

4. **Low systolic** and **low diastolic** numbers with a **rapid Heart rate**, indicating "empty heat" exists. In this case, one must build the cool, moist, nourishing aspect of the body.

More generally, the Liver has 600 physiological functions, of which one is to help the body cope with life's emotional stresses. Another of the Liver's functions is to drive the blood and energy freely through the body in a relaxed fashion. In other words, if the Liver is functioning well, the blood vessels are relaxed and stable. In addition, the Liver "nourishes" Heart function (the Heart has an important role in high blood pressure; however, the Heart derives much of its function from the Liver).

An example follows: one experiences long-lasting emotional stress and eventually the Liver starts to break down, leading to decreased Heart function. The blood vessels begin to contract, over time becoming rigid. With the same volume of blood in now inelastic blood vessels, the pressure increases hence, high blood pressure.

Given that one of the Liver's 600 functions is to purify the bloodstream, reducing or eliminating the intake of toxic chemicals is very important as part of a larger strategy to resolve high blood pressure. Given that the Heart and Liver are likely involved at least to some degree, it is important to exercise gently (under the supervision of your doctor) for at least 30 minutes four times weekly, thus increasing circulation, soothing the

Heart and Liver and stimulating increased circulation throughout the body, which allows the blood vessels to relax.

As you can see with this particular health problem, there is an underlying cause. The key to success in treating these problems lies in addressing the underlying issue described above to eliminate the problem over the long term. To speed Acupuncture and/or Chinese Herbal Medicine results, it is recommended one minimally reduce or eliminate the intake of caffeine, deep-fried foods, dairy, sugar, preservatives in food, chemicals in food and municipal tap water (which most often contains chlorine and fluoride, considered by many as dangerous chemicals).

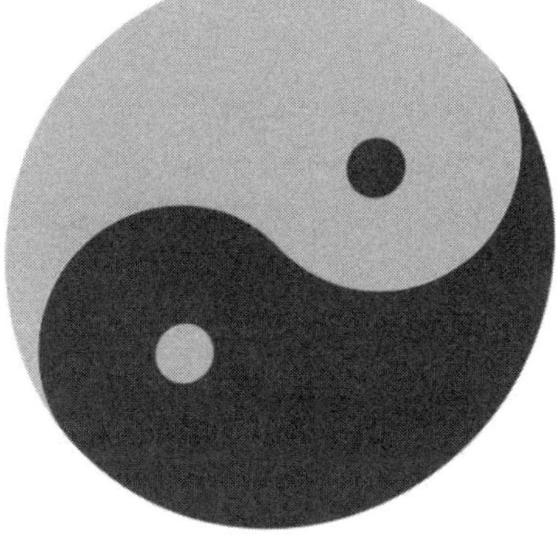

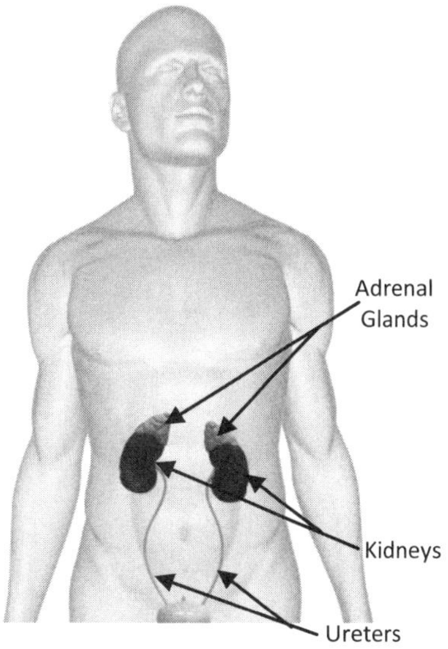

Hot Flashes

Hot flashes have many potential causes, however what follows are the basic mechanics. The Kidney/Adrenal system is the root of the "yin" and the "yang" of the body. The yin is the cool, moist and nourishing aspect of the body (for example, the amniotic fluid around the baby); whereas yang is hot, moving and invigorating (an example of yang gone "awry" is a woman having a hot flash).

When the yin is deficient, the yang can "rise" (heat rises) to the surface of the body, causing an intense sensation of heat and possibly perspiration.

As you can see with this particular health problem, there is an underlying cause. The key to success in treating these problems lies in addressing the underlying issue described above to eliminate the problem over the long term. To speed Acupuncture and/or Chinese Herbal Medicine results, it is recommended one minimally reduce or eliminate the intake of caffeine, deep-fried foods, dairy, sugar, preservatives in food, chemicals in food and municipal tap water (which most often contains chlorine and fluoride, considered by many as dangerous chemicals).

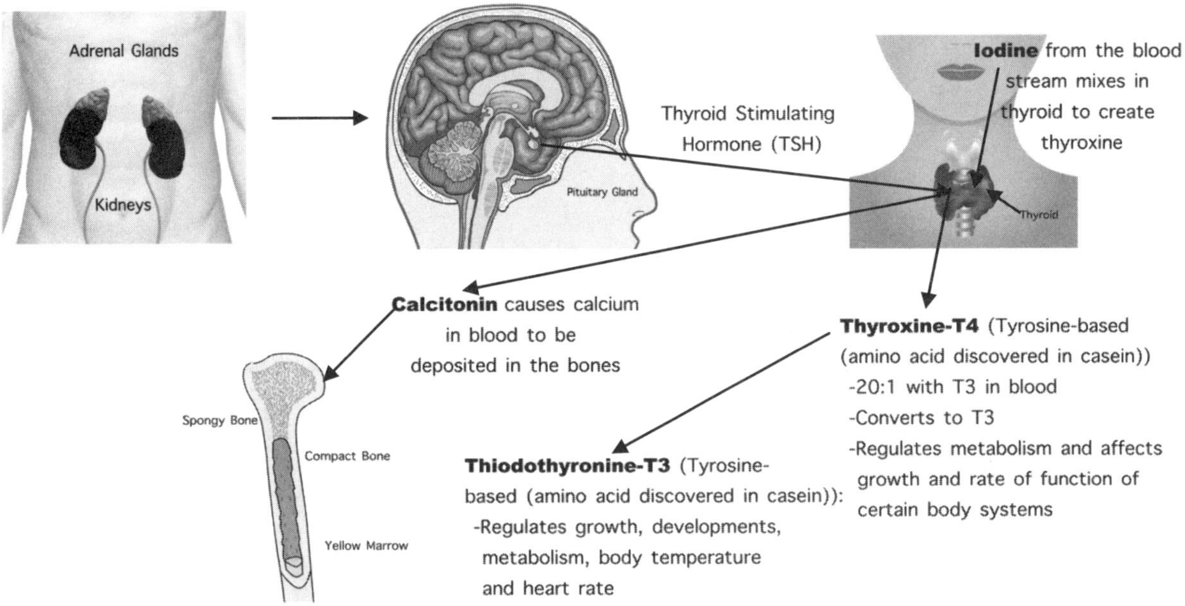

Hypothyroid (under-active thyroid)/ Hyperthyroid (over-active thyroid)

Thyroid imbalances have many potential causes, however what follows are the basic mechanics. The Kidney/Adrenal system produces raw materials that stimulate glands (including the thyroid) to produce hormones that drive the endocrine system (the network of glands that produce secretions that drive many bodily functions). Too much or too little Kidney/Adrenal function can cause thyroid imbalances. The Thyroid is simply a superficial aspect of the problem.

Overall, the Thyroid controls the body's use of energy, the body's production of proteins and the body's sensitivity to other hormones in the following manner:

The Kidney/Adrenal system stimulates Pituitary gland function; in turn, the Pituitary gland releases Thyroid Stimulating Hormone (TSH) to the Thyroid, generating much of its function. Iodine from the blood stream is used by the Thyroid to create Thyroxin (known as T4, which regulates metabolism, growth and rate of function of other body systems); eventually T4 converts in the bloodstream into Triiodothyronine (known as T3, which regulates growth, development, metabolism, body temperature and heart rate). The Thyroid also releases Calcitonin, which helps deposit calcium in the bloodstream into bone tissue.

In both Hypothyroid and Hyperthyroid conditions, one must regulate Thyroid function by normalizing the appropriate out-of-balance variable from the description above. Certain thyroid medications may cause the thyroid to atrophy: taking these medications for a period of time may cause the thyroid to shrink and lose function due to its inactivity. The longer period of time that one takes these medications, the less chance for the thyroid to recover, it seems.

As you can see with this particular health problem, there is an underlying cause. The key to success in treating these problems lies in addressing the underlying issue described above to eliminate the problem over the long term. To speed Acupuncture and/or Chinese Herbal Medicine results, it is recommended one minimally reduce or eliminate the intake of caffeine, deep-fried foods, dairy, sugar, preservatives in food, chemicals in food and municipal tap water (which most often contains chlorine and fluoride, considered by many as dangerous chemicals).

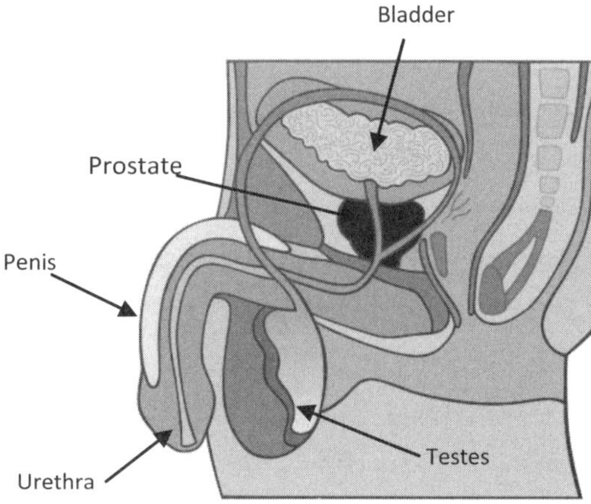

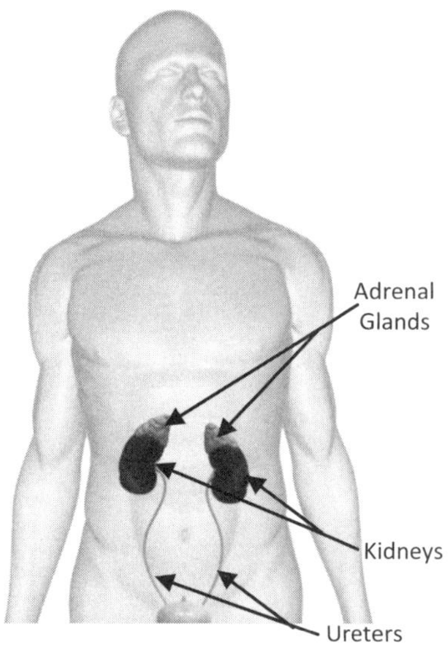

Impotence

Impotence has many potential causes, however what follows are the basic mechanics. The Kidney/Adrenal system produces raw materials for the production of hormones (for example, testosterone) that the body uses to control many functions, including reproductive organ function.

Two basic aspects of the Kidney/Adrenal system are the "yin" and the "yang." The yin is cool, moist, and nourishing (example: the amniotic fluid around a baby). On the other hand, yang is hot, invigorating and moving (example: yang's driving force moving into the male genitals causing an erection). All of the reproductive hormones have either more yin or more yang properties for example, testosterone has very yang properties that are vital to drive the male reproductive system. Impotence may be caused by what is called "Kidney yang deficiency."

As you can see with this particular health problem, there is an underlying cause. The key to success in treating these problems lies in addressing the underlying issue described above to eliminate the problem over the long term. To speed Acupuncture and/or Chinese Herbal Medicine results, it is recommended one minimally reduce or eliminate the intake of caffeine, deep-fried foods, dairy, sugar, preservatives in food, chemicals in food and municipal tap water (which most often contains chlorine and fluoride, considered by many as dangerous chemicals).

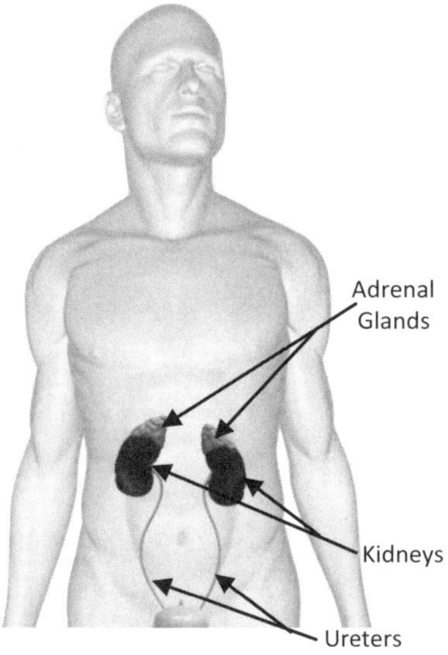

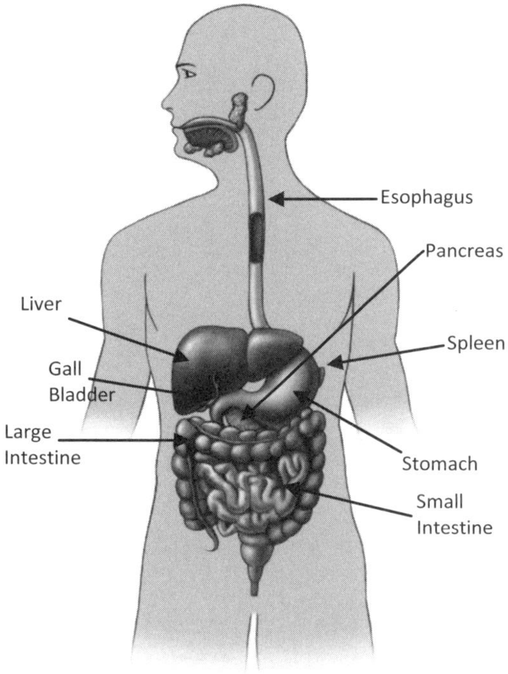

Incontinence-bowel

Bowel incontinence has many potential causes, however what follows are the basic mechanics. The Kidney/Adrenal system is in charge of opening and closing the lower "orifices" (the urethra for urination and the anus for the bowels)[5].

When the Kidney/Adrenal system is working normally, it causes the urethra and anus to "open" and "close" at appropriate times; conversely, if the Kidney/ Adrenal system lose function, the urethra and/or anus may open involuntarily, causing bowel or urinary "leakage."

As you can see with this particular health problem, there is an underlying cause. The key to success in treating these problems lies in addressing the underlying issue described above to eliminate the problem over the long term. To speed Acupuncture and/or Chinese Herbal Medicine results, it is recommended one minimally reduce or

---

[5] Maciocia, Giovanni, *The Foundations of Chinese Medicine*, New York: Churchhill Livingstone, 1989. 498p.

eliminate the intake of caffeine, deep-fried foods, dairy, sugar, preservatives in food, chemicals in food and municipal tap water (which most often contains chlorine and fluoride, considered by many as dangerous chemicals).

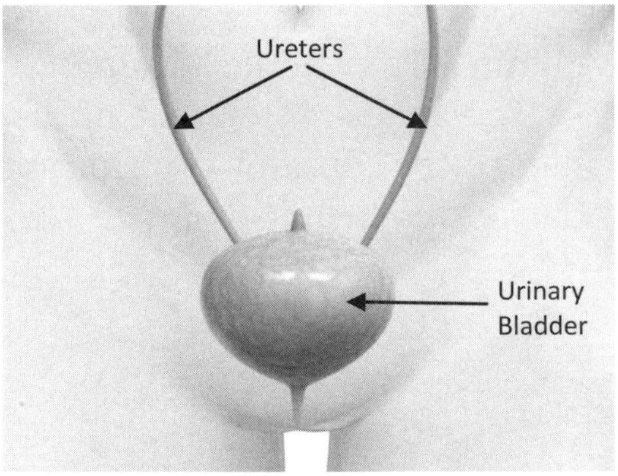

Incontinence-urinary

Urinary incontinence has many potential causes, however what follows are the basic mechanics. The Kidney/Adrenal system is in charge of opening and closing the lower "orifices" (the urethra for urination and the anus for the bowels)[6].

When the Kidney/Adrenal system is working normally, it causes the urethra and anus to "open" and "close" at appropriate times; conversely, if the Kidney/ Adrenal system lose function, the urethra and/or anus may open involuntarily, causing bowel or urinary "leakage."

As you can see with this particular health problem, there is an underlying cause. The key to success in treating these problems lies in addressing the underlying issue described above to eliminate the problem over the long term. To speed Acupuncture and/or Chinese Herbal Medicine results, it is recommended one minimally reduce or eliminate the intake of caffeine, deep-fried foods, dairy, sugar, preservatives in food, chemicals in food and municipal tap water (which most often contains chlorine and fluoride, considered by many as dangerous chemicals).

---

[6] Maciocia, Giovanni, *The Foundations of Chinese Medicine*, New York: Churchhill Livingstone, 1989. 498p.

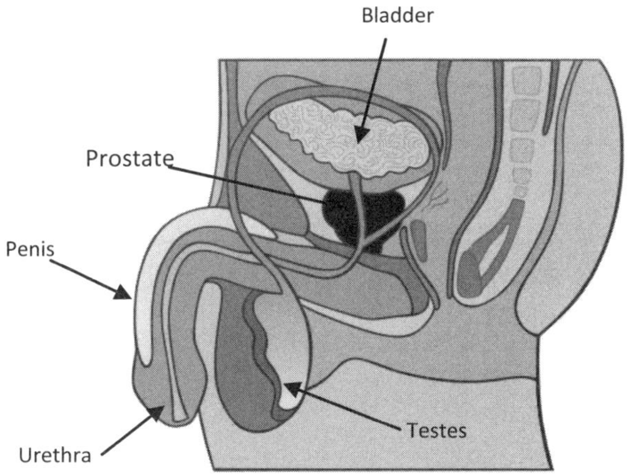

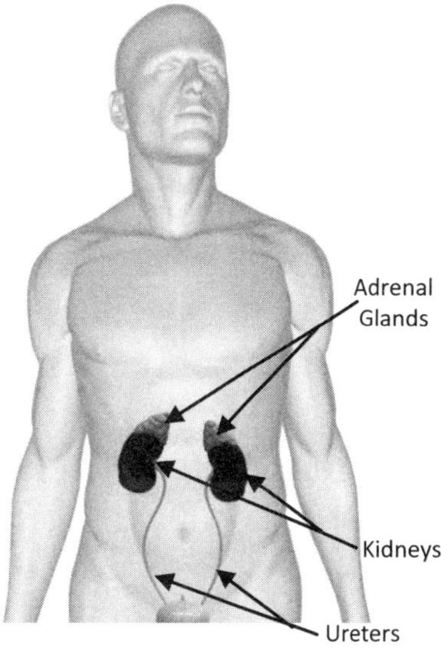

Infertility-Men

Male infertility has many potential causes, however what follows are the basic mechanics. The Kidney/Adrenal system produces raw materials necessary for the production of hormones that govern male reproductive system function, including the ability to produce adequate amounts of properly functioning and "motile" (a biology term referring an ability something has to move itself) sperm.

Some men have high quantities of toxic material in the body that spread to the reproductive organs, causing infertility. In such cases, one must detoxify the body, which may be done with Acupuncture and/or Chinese Herbal Medicine.

Another possible cause of male infertility may be what is called "Kidney yang deficiency." Two basic aspects of the Kidney/Adrenal system are "yin" and "yang." Yin is cool, moist, and nourishing (an example of this would be the amniotic fluid around a baby in a woman's womb). On the other hand, yang is hot, invigorating and moving (an example of this in a man's body is yang's driving force behind the production of and motility of sperm). All of the reproductive hormones have either more yin or more yang properties; for example, testosterone has very yang properties that are vital to drive the male reproductive system.

As you can see with this particular health problem, there is an underlying cause. The key to success in treating these problems lies in addressing the underlying issue described above to eliminate the problem over the long term. To speed Acupuncture and/or Chinese Herbal Medicine results, it is recommended one minimally reduce or eliminate the intake of caffeine, deep-fried foods, dairy, sugar, preservatives in food, chemicals in food and municipal tap water (which most often contains chlorine and fluoride, considered by many as dangerous chemicals). One very good substitute for butter that increases fertility in both men and women is "ghee" (clarified butter).

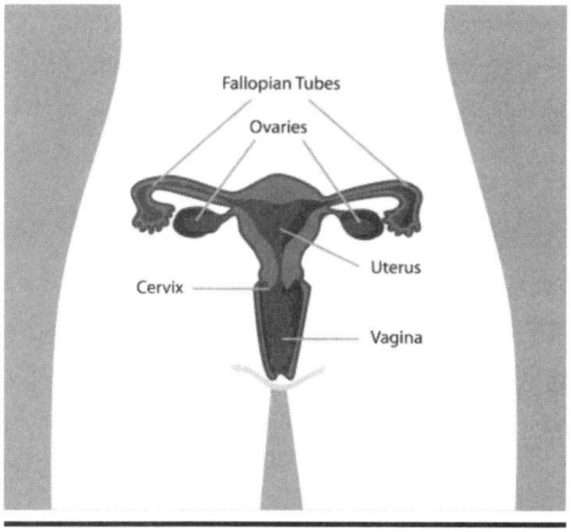

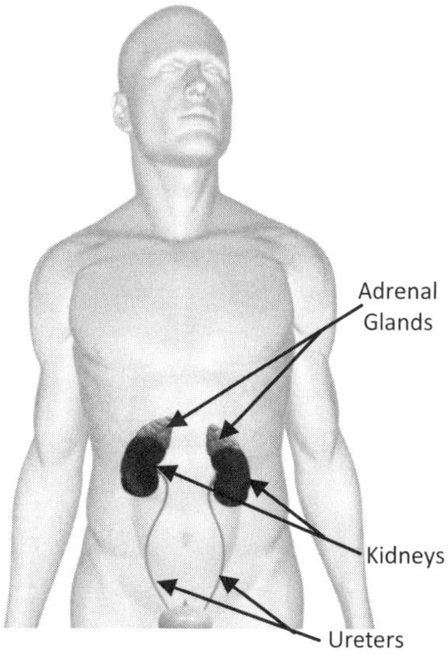

Infertility-Women

Female infertility has many potential causes, however what follows are the basic mechanics. The Kidney/Adrenal system produces raw materials necessary for the production of hormones that govern female reproductive system function, including hormones that ensure plentiful, fertile eggs exist and move freely within the fallopian tube.

Four potential causes of infertility follow:

1. Lack of Kidney/Adrenal system function can lead to inadequate raw materials necessary for the production of reproductive hormones, thus leading to infertility. Two basic aspects of the Kidney/Adrenal system are "yin" and "yang." Yin is cool, moist, and nourishing (an example of this would be the amniotic fluid around a baby in a woman's womb). On the other hand, yang is hot, invigorating and moving (an example of yang gone "awry" would be a woman having a hot flash). Female reproductive hormones have either more yin or more yang properties for example, estrogen (which helps prepare the body for and maintain a pregnancy)

may have more yang properties and progesterone (which helps prepare the uterus for receiving and nourishing a fertilized egg) may have more yin properties. Reproductive hormone balance (therefore Kidney yin and yang balance) is critical for conception and a full-term pregnancy.

2. If a woman's body does not manufacture enough blood (which carries reproductive hormones to those areas of the body involved with conception and pregnancy) to nourish the inside lining of the uterus, the uterus may not be able to accept the attachment of, or even sustain, a fertilized egg, much less allow the baby to fully develop.

3. "Cold-Womb Syndrome" is a condition wherein cold may be "trapped" in the uterus, making it inhospitable for a fertilized egg. This phenomenon may be caused in some cases by a woman walking around unclothed in a cold environment after sexual activity.

4. Excess toxic material in the body and/or reproductive system may create a dangerous environment in the uterus for the attachment of a fertilized egg.

As you can see with this particular health problem, there is an underlying cause. The key to success in treating these problems lies in addressing the underlying issue described above to eliminate the problem over the long term. To speed Acupuncture and/or Chinese Herbal Medicine results, it is recommended one minimally reduce or eliminate the intake of caffeine, deep-fried foods, dairy, sugar, preservatives in food, chemicals in food and municipal tap water (which most often contains chlorine and fluoride, considered by many as dangerous chemicals). One very good substitute for butter that can be helpful for fertility in both men and women is "ghee" (clarified butter).

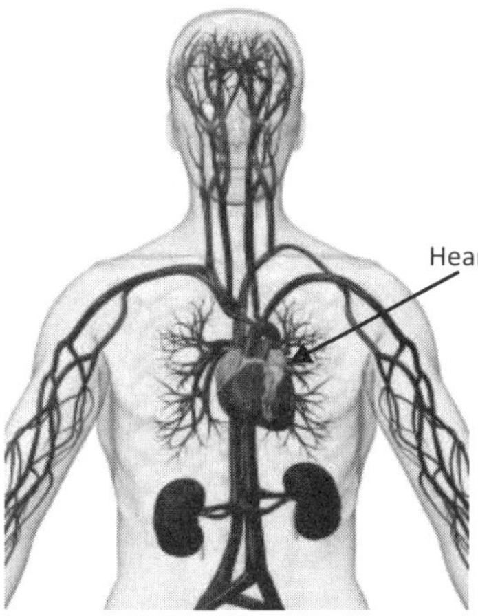

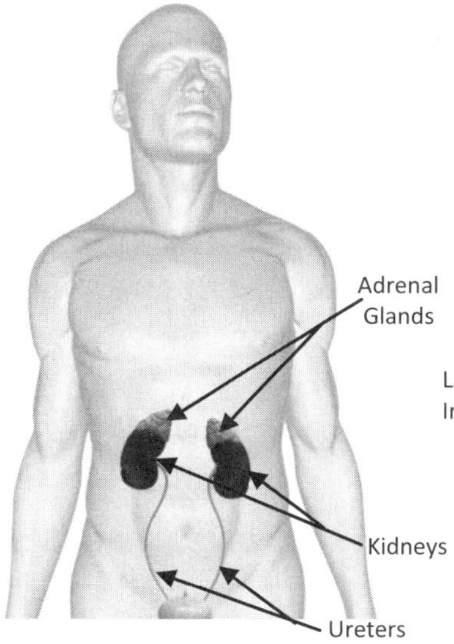

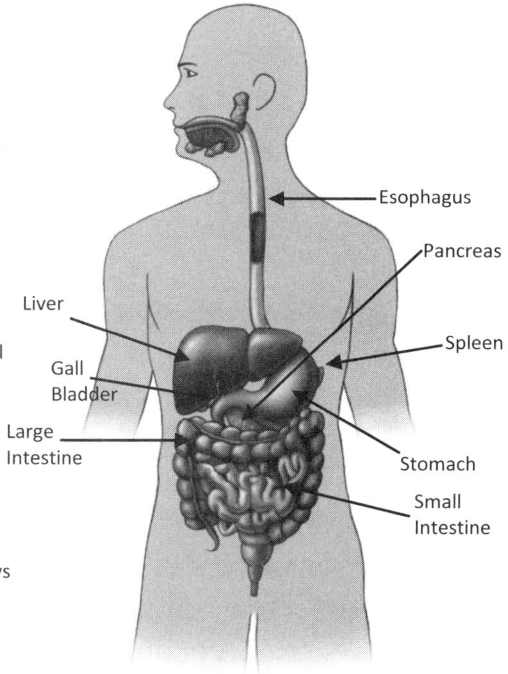

Insomnia-Difficulty falling asleep at night

There are many potential causes and types of insomnia, however what follows are the basic mechanics. When the mind becomes overactive, often times it may cause one to have difficulty falling asleep. There are potentially three organ systems that may be involved that may throw the involved sleep hormones out of balance:

1. Spleen/Pancreatic system malfunction may cause difficulty falling asleep due to over-thinking.

2. Heart malfunction may cause difficulty falling asleep due to anxiety.

3. Kidney/Adrenal system imbalances may cause difficulty falling asleep. The Kidney/Adrenal system is the root of the "yin" and the "yang" of the body. Yin is the cool, moist and nourishing aspect of the body (for example the amniotic fluid around the baby); whereas yang is warming,

moving and invigorating (an example of yang gone awry would be a woman having a hot flash). Nighttime is the most yin time of the day; a Kidney/Adrenal system breakdown may cause the yang to "rise" and stimulate the function of the mind, which should be calm in the evening.

As you can see with this particular health problem, there is an underlying cause. The key to success in treating these problems lies in addressing the underlying issue described above to eliminate the problem over the long term. To speed Acupuncture and/or Chinese Herbal Medicine results, it is recommended one minimally reduce or eliminate the intake of caffeine, deep-fried foods, dairy, sugar, preservatives in food, chemicals in food and municipal tap water (which most often contains chlorine and fluoride, considered by many as dangerous chemicals).

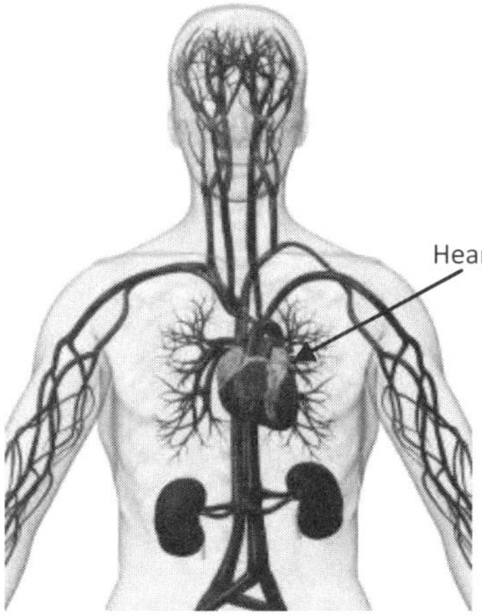

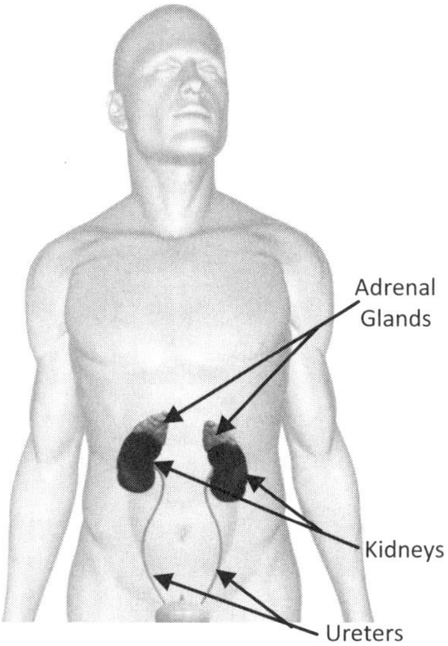

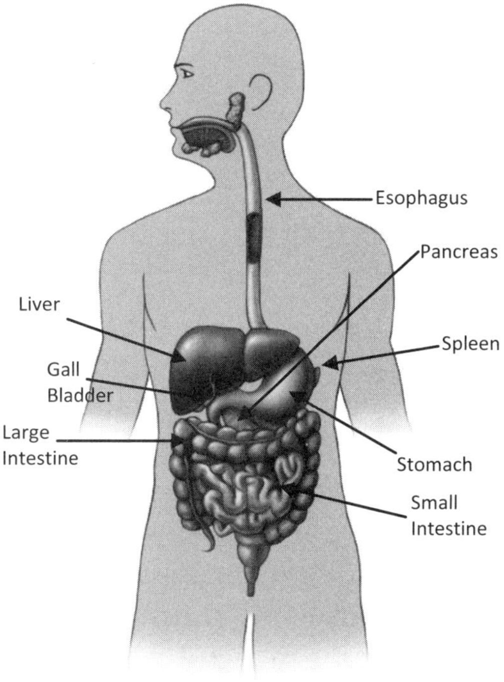

Insomnia-Waking in the middle of the night

There are many potential causes and types of insomnia, however what follows are the basic mechanics. When the mind becomes overactive, often times it may cause one to wake in the middle of the night. There are four potential organ systems that may be involved that may throw the hormones necessary for sleep out of balance:

1. Spleen/Pancreatic system malfunction may cause one to wake in the middle of the night due to over-thinking.

2. Heart malfunction may cause one to wake in the middle of the night due to anxiety.

3. Liver inflammation may cause one to wake in the middle of the night.

4. Kidney/Adrenal system imbalances may cause one to wake in the middle of the night, either due to nighttime urination and/or hormonal imbalances. The Kidney/Adrenal system is the root of the "yin" and the "yang" of the body. Yin is the cool, moist and nourishing aspect of the body (for example the amniotic fluid around the baby); whereas yang is warming, moving and invigorating (an example of yang gone awry would be a woman having a hot flash). Nighttime is the most yin time of the day; a Kidney/Adrenal system breakdown may cause the yang to "rise" and stimulate the function of the mind, which is calm in the evening under normal circumstances.

As you can see with this particular health problem, there is an underlying cause. The key to success in treating these problems lies in addressing the underlying issue described above to eliminate the problem over the long term. To speed Acupuncture and/or Chinese Herbal Medicine results, it is recommended one minimally reduce or eliminate the intake of caffeine, deep-fried foods, dairy, sugar, preservatives in food, chemicals in food and municipal tap water (which most often contains chlorine and fluoride, considered by many as dangerous chemicals).

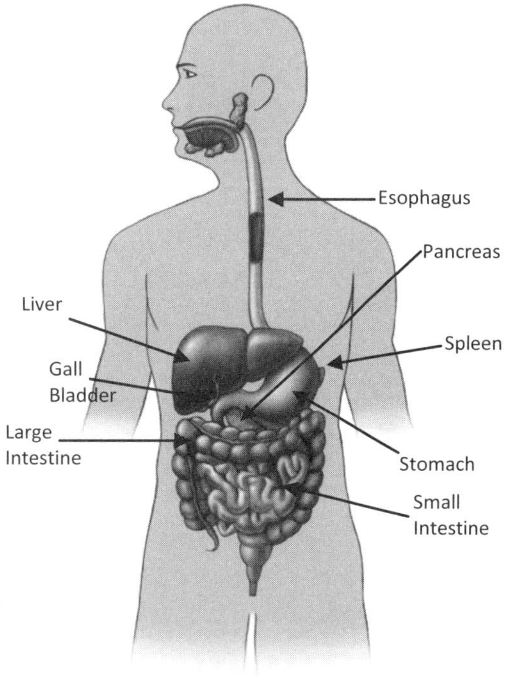

Insomnia-Waking in the morning earlier than normal

There are many potential causes and types of insomnia, however what follows are the basic mechanics. The Liver performs 600 physiological functions, one of which is to allow an individual adapt to the mental and emotional stresses of life. A loss of Liver function, given its relationship to mental function and stress, may cause the mind to become active earlier in the morning than normal, thus awakening one.

Given that another of the Liver's 600 functions is to purify the bloodstream, reducing or eliminating the intake of toxic chemicals is very important as part of a larger strategy to resolve depression. It is also important to exercise vigorously (to a point of perspiration) for at least 30 minutes four times weekly, thus increasing Liver circulation, soothing the Liver and stimulating increased circulation throughout the body, which allows the body to detoxify at least to a small degree.

As you can see with this particular health problem, there is an underlying cause. The key to success in treating these problems lies in addressing the underlying issue described above to eliminate the problem over the long term. To speed Acupuncture and/or Chinese Herbal Medicine results, it is recommended one minimally reduce or eliminate the intake of caffeine, deep-fried foods, dairy, sugar, preservatives in food, chemicals in food and municipal tap water (which most often contains chlorine and fluoride, considered by many as dangerous chemicals).

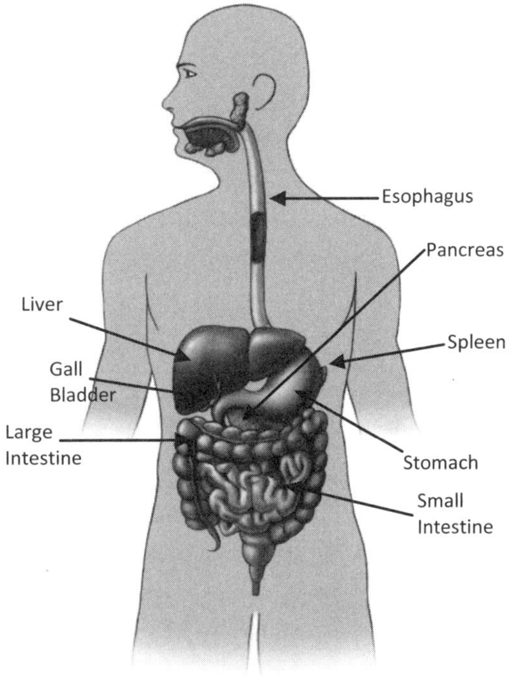

Irritability

Excessive or inappropriate irritability has many potential causes, however what follows are the basic mechanics. Thousands of years ago, physicians in China began to explore the nature of human emotion and discovered a direct link between emotion and the organ system. Having helped many people resolve emotional imbalances over the years, we've found the following to be accurate from the point of view of the physical body (obviously many factors exist in life that may trigger bodily malfunction which, in turn, could then trigger an emotional response). What is described below is the relationship between the emotions and physical body.

The Liver has 600 physiological functions, one of which is to help the body adapt to the mental and emotional stresses of life. In other words, if one's Liver is functioning at a high level, stress entering one's life has no physical effect; however, if one's Liver isn't functioning well, stress can have a negative effect on the body.

Liver malfunction can cause a person to experience excessive or inappropriate anger, irritability, frustration, impatience, and/or depression. For example, a person with multiple emotional stresses over many years may experience suppressed Liver function. Then, the loss of a loved one could cause Liver function to drop dramatically, and the person could then begin to experience excessive or inappropriate irritability. On the other hand, a well-functioning Liver will cause one to be emotionally even and generally happy.

Irritability may be caused by a breakdown in Liver function, not simply an imbalance in brain chemistry (the typical Western Medical view of this particular condition). Ironically, addressing only the brain chemistry with medication often leads to further difficulty resolving the problem as shown here: if one takes a medication for irritability (which may be caused by a Liver imbalance) and that medication reduces Liver function (the Liver, in its capacity as a blood purifier, will attempt to eliminate the chemical from the body), it makes it more difficult to treat the irritability. This explains why a person may take a medication their entire life.....and the irritability never fully resolves!

Given that one of the Liver's 600 functions is to purify the bloodstream, reducing or eliminating the intake of toxic chemicals is very important as part of a larger strategy to resolve irritability. It is also important to exercise vigorously (to a point of perspiration) for at least 30 minutes four times weekly, thus increasing Liver circulation, soothing the Liver and stimulating increased circulation throughout the body, which allows the body to detoxify at least to a small degree.

As you can see with this particular health problem, there is an underlying cause. The key to success in treating these problems lies in addressing the underlying issue described above to eliminate the problem over the long term. To speed Acupuncture and/or Chinese

Herbal Medicine results, it is recommended one minimally reduce or eliminate the intake of caffeine, deep-fried foods, dairy, sugar, preservatives in food, chemicals in food and municipal tap water (which most often contains chlorine and fluoride, considered by many as dangerous chemicals).

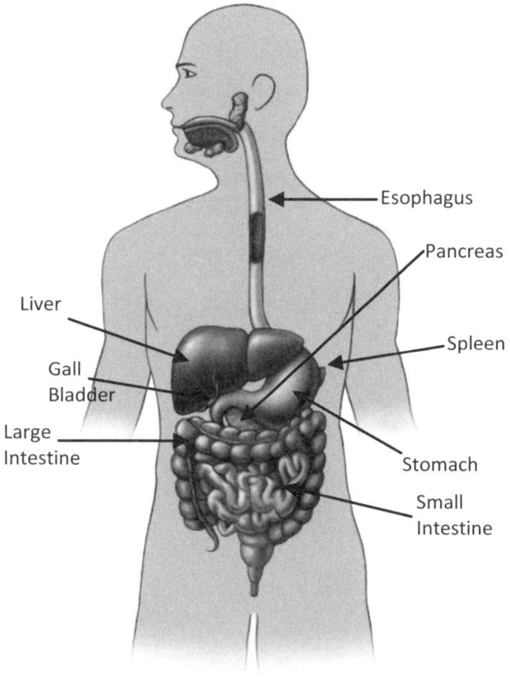

Irritable Bowel Syndrome

Irritable Bowel Syndrome may be caused by spasms in the Small and/or Large Intestine. The Liver performs 600 physiological functions, one of which is helping one adapt to the mental and emotional stresses of life; under excessive emotional and/or chemical stress, the Liver (which has a direct connection to the intestinal tract) may negatively affect the Large and/or Small Intestine. A breakdown in Liver function may cause a problem of weakened metabolism of food, constriction around along the intestinal tract and/or spasmodic muscle contractions along the intestinal tract, leading to digestive irregularity, constipation, diarrhea, gas and/or bloating.

Given that one of the Liver's 600 functions is to purify the bloodstream, reducing or eliminating the intake of toxic chemicals is very important as part of a larger strategy to resolve irritability. It is also important to exercise vigorously (to a point of perspiration) for at least 30 minutes four times weekly, thus increasing Liver circulation, soothing the Liver and stimulating increased circulation throughout the body, which allows the body to detoxify at least to a small degree.

As you can see with this particular health problem, there is an underlying cause. The key to success in treating these problems lies in addressing the underlying issue described above to eliminate the problem over the long term. To speed Acupuncture and/or Chinese Herbal Medicine results, it is recommended one minimally reduce or eliminate the intake of caffeine, deep-fried foods, dairy, sugar, preservatives in food, chemicals in food and municipal tap water (which most often contains chlorine and fluoride, considered by many as dangerous chemicals).

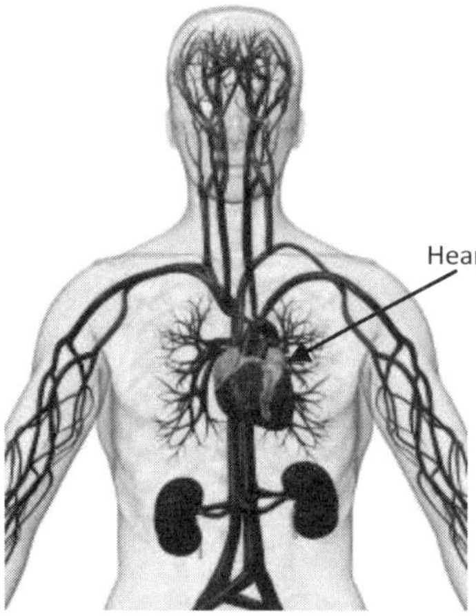

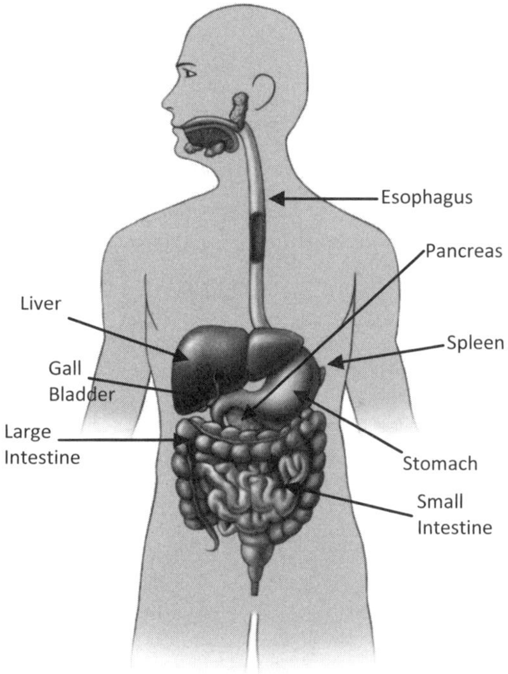

Low Blood Pressure

Low blood pressure has several potential causes, however what follows are the basic mechanics. Blood pressure is obviously regulated by the Heart, but also the Liver, and, to a certain degree, the Kidney/Adrenal system.

Low Blood Pressure

Generally, the successful treatment of low blood pressure involves building the affected organ systems' function until they are functioning normally as well as taking the following into account.

Categories of blood pressure problems:[7]

1. **High systolic** and **high diastolic** numbers with a **high pulse rate**, indicating "heat" and/or toxicity is trapped internally.

[7] Chang, Jimmy Wei-Yen and Brinkman, Marcus, *Pulsesynergy: A Pulse Diagnosis Manual*, 1995. 166p.

2. **Low systolic** and **low diastolic** numbers with a **slow pulse rate**, indicating the hot, invigorating aspect of the body is depleted. In such as case one must increase internal "heat" and increase circulation dramatically.

3. **High systolic** and **normal to high diastolic** numbers with a **slow pulse rate**, indicating blood circulation is stagnating and that "empty heat" exists. In such a case one must increase blood circulation dramatically and build the cool, moist, nourishing aspect of the body.

4. **Low systolic** and **low diastolic** numbers with a **rapid Heart rate**, indicating "empty heat" exists. In this case, one must build the cool, moist, nourishing aspect of the body.

Given that one of the Liver's 600 functions is to purify the bloodstream, reducing or eliminating the intake of toxic chemicals is very important as part of a larger strategy to resolve high blood pressure. Given that the Heart and Liver are likely involved at least to some degree, it is important to exercise gently (under the supervision of your doctor) for at least 30 minutes four times weekly, thus increasing circulation, soothing the Heart and Liver and stimulating increased circulation throughout the body, which allows the blood vessels to relax.

As you can see with this particular health problem, there is an underlying cause. The key to success in treating these problems lies in addressing the underlying issue described above to eliminate the problem over the long term. To speed Acupuncture and/or Chinese Herbal Medicine results, it is recommended one minimally reduce or eliminate the intake of caffeine, deep-fried foods, dairy, sugar, preservatives in food, chemicals in food and municipal tap water (which most often contains chlorine and fluoride, considered by many as dangerous chemicals).

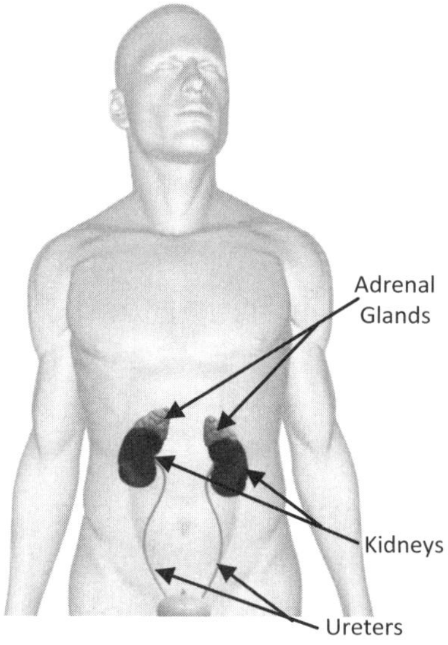

Memory: Long-Term Memory Loss

Long-term memory loss has many potential causes, however what follows are the basic mechanics. The Kidney/Adrenal system is responsible for many bodily functions, including long-term memory.

Long-term memory loss may be caused by Kidney/Adrenal system malfunction or a head injury.

As you can see with this particular health problem, there is an underlying cause. The key to success in treating these problems lies in addressing the underlying issue described above to eliminate the problem over the long term. To speed Acupuncture and/or Chinese Herbal Medicine results, it is recommended one minimally reduce or eliminate the intake of caffeine, deep-fried foods, dairy, sugar, preservatives in food, chemicals in food and municipal tap water (which most often contains chlorine and fluoride, considered by many as dangerous chemicals).

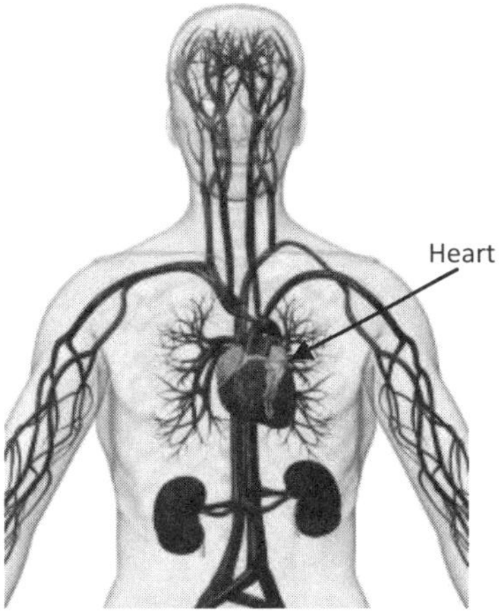

Memory:
Short-Term Memory Loss

Short-term memory loss has many potential causes, however what follows are the basic mechanics. The Heart governs the "mind" or mental faculties of an individual. When Heart function drops it may cause short-term memory loss. Obviously, head injuries may also contribute to memory loss.

As you can see with this particular health problem, there is an underlying cause. The key to success in treating these problems lies in addressing the underlying issue described above to eliminate the problem over the long term. To speed Acupuncture and/or Chinese Herbal Medicine results, it is recommended one minimally reduce or eliminate the intake of caffeine, deep-fried foods, dairy, sugar, preservatives in food, chemicals in food and municipal tap water (which most often contains chlorine and fluoride, considered by many as dangerous chemicals).

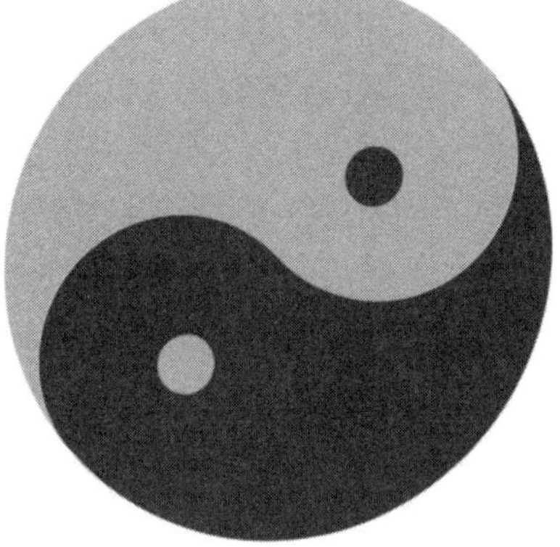

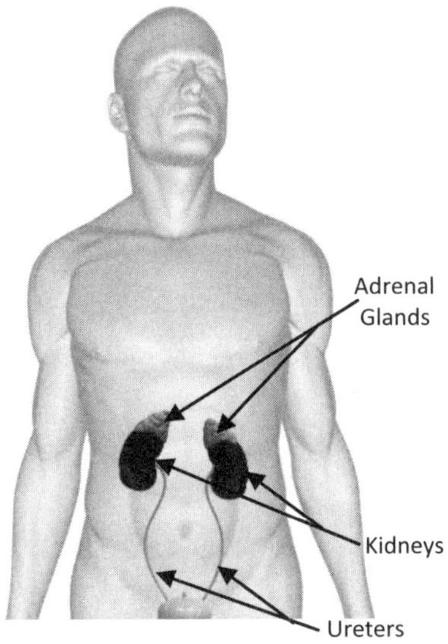

Menopausal Hot Flashes

Menopausal hot flashes have many potential causes, however what follows are the basic mechanics. Lack of Kidney/Adrenal system function can lead to inadequate raw materials necessary for the production of reproductive hormones, thus leading to hot flashes.

Two basic aspects of the Kidney/Adrenal system are "yin" and "yang." Yin is cool, moist, and nourishing (an example of this would be the amniotic fluid around a baby in a woman's womb). On the other hand, yang is hot, invigorating and moving (an example of yang gone "awry" would be a woman having a hot flash). Female reproductive hormones have either more yin or more yang properties for example, estrogen (which helps prepare the body for and maintain a pregnancy) may have more yang properties and progesterone (which helps prepare the uterus for receiving and nourishing a fertilized egg) may have more yin properties. Reproductive hormone balance (therefore Kidney yin and yang balance) is critical for normal body temperature.

When such hormones slip out of balance, many symptoms, including hot flashes, may result. The yin may become deficient, causing the yang to "rise" to the surface of the body, causing an intense sensation of heat and possibly perspiration.

As you can see with this particular health problem, there is an underlying cause. The key to success in treating these problems lies in addressing the underlying issue described above to eliminate the problem over the long term. To speed Acupuncture and/or Chinese Herbal Medicine results, it is recommended one minimally reduce or eliminate the intake of caffeine, deep-fried foods, dairy, sugar, preservatives in food, chemicals in food and municipal tap water (which most often contains chlorine and fluoride, considered by many as dangerous chemicals).

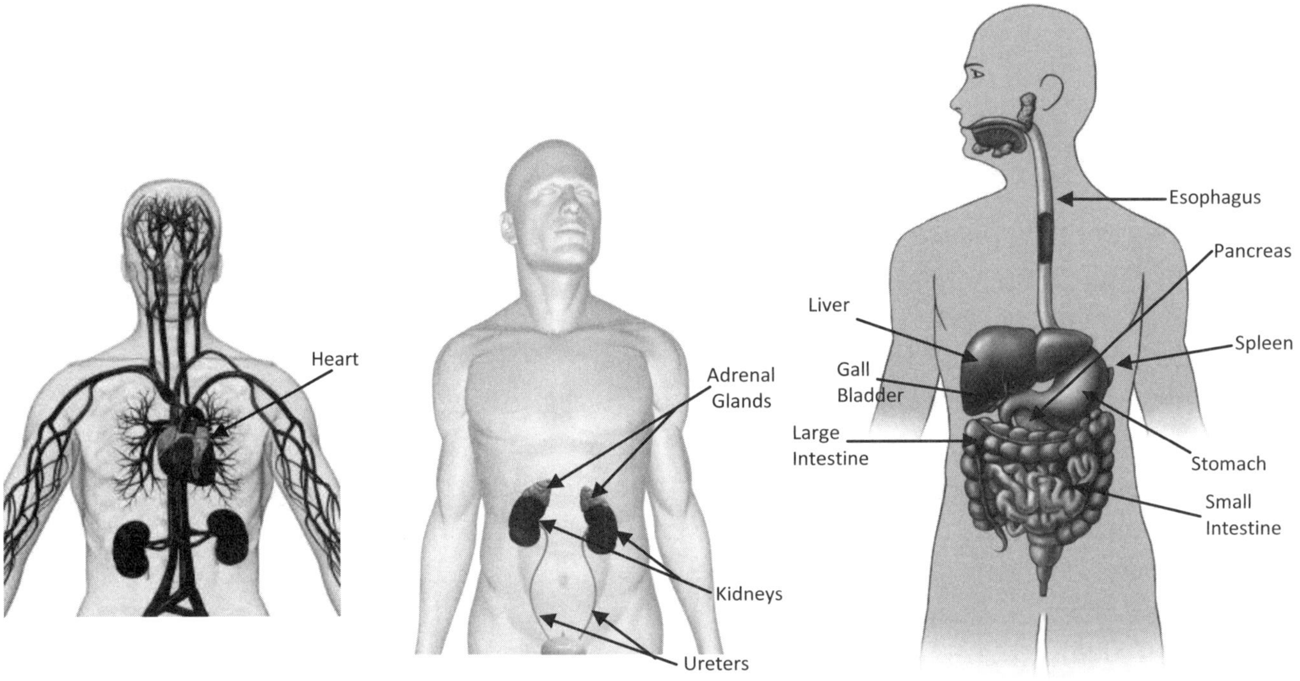

Menopausal Insomnia-Difficulty Falling Asleep at Night

There are many potential causes and types of insomnia, however what follows are the basic mechanics. When the mind becomes overactive, often times it may cause one to have difficulty falling asleep. There are potentially three organ systems that may be involved, thus throwing the hormones necessary for normal sleep out of balance:

1. Spleen/Pancreatic system malfunction may cause difficulty falling asleep due to over-thinking.

2. Heart malfunction may cause difficulty falling asleep due to anxiety.

3. Kidney/Adrenal system imbalances may cause difficulty falling asleep, especially in cases of menopause. The Kidney/Adrenal system is the root of the "yin" and the "yang" of the body and produces the raw materials for hormones (which themselves have more yin or yang qualities)

necessary for adequate sleep. Yin is the cool, moist and nourishing aspect of the body (for example the amniotic fluid around the baby); whereas yang is warming, moving and invigorating (an example of yang gone awry would be a woman having a hot flash). Nighttime is the most yin time of the day; a Kidney/Adrenal system breakdown may cause the yang to "rise" and stimulate the function of the mind, which is calm in the evening under normal circumstances.

As you can see with this particular health problem, there is an underlying cause. The key to success in treating these problems lies in addressing the underlying issue described above to eliminate the problem over the long term. To speed Acupuncture and/or Chinese Herbal Medicine results, it is recommended one minimally reduce or eliminate the intake of caffeine, deep-fried foods, dairy, sugar, preservatives in food, chemicals in food and municipal tap water (which most often contains chlorine and fluoride, considered by many as dangerous chemicals).

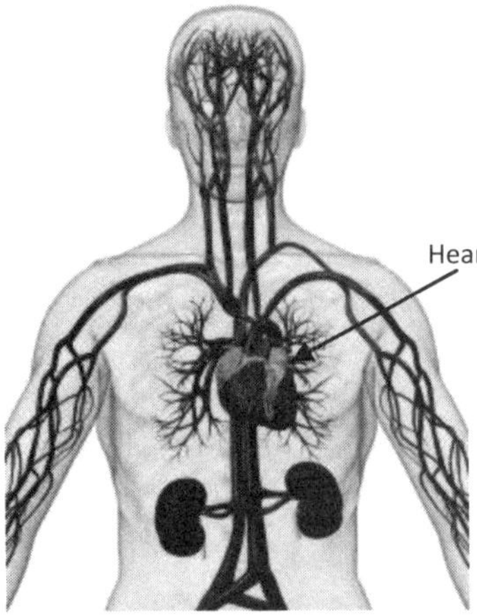

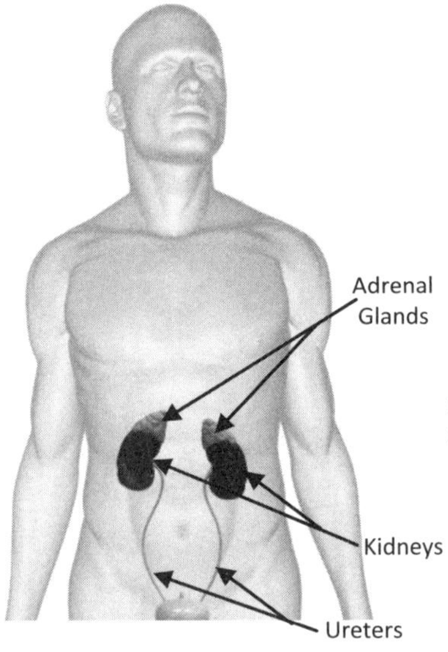

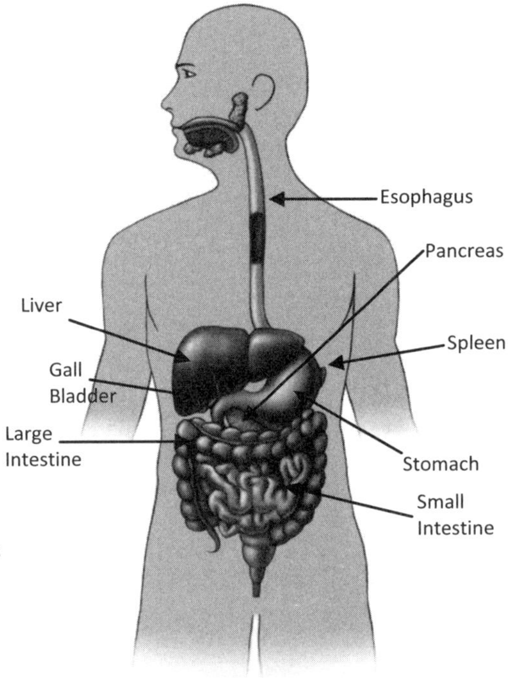

Menopausal Insomnia-Waking at Night

There are many potential causes and types of insomnia, however what follows are the basic mechanics. When the mind becomes overactive, often times it may cause one to wake in the middle of the night. There are four potential organ systems that may be involved, thus throwing the hormones necessary for normal sleep out of balance:

1. Spleen/Pancreatic system malfunction may cause one to wake in the middle of the night due to over-thinking.

2. Heart malfunction may cause one to wake in the middle of the night due to anxiety.

3. Liver inflammation may cause one to wake in the middle of the night.

4. Kidney/Adrenal system imbalances may cause one to wake in the middle of the night, either due to nighttime urination and/or hormonal imbalances common in menopause. The Kidney/Adrenal system is the root of the "yin" and the "yang" of the body. Yin is the cool, moist and nourishing aspect of the body (for example the amniotic fluid around the baby); whereas yang is warming, moving and invigorating (an example of yang gone awry would be a woman having a hot flash). Nighttime is the most yin time of the day; a Kidney/Adrenal system breakdown may cause the yang to "rise" and stimulate the function of the mind, which is calm in the evening under normal circumstances.

As you can see with this particular health problem, there is an underlying cause. The key to success in treating these problems lies in addressing the underlying issue described above to eliminate the problem over the long term. To speed Acupuncture and/or Chinese Herbal Medicine results, it is recommended one minimally reduce or eliminate the intake of caffeine, deep-fried foods, dairy, sugar, preservatives in food, chemicals in food and municipal tap water (which most often contains chlorine and fluoride, considered by many as dangerous chemicals).

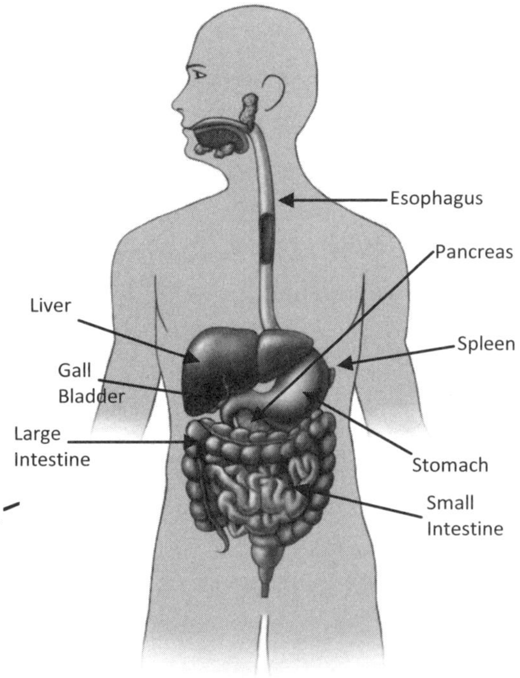

Menopausal Insomnia-Waking Earlier in the Morning Than Usual

There are many potential causes and types of insomnia, however what follows are the basic mechanics. The Liver performs 600 physiological functions, one of which is to allow an individual adapt to the mental and emotional stresses of life. A loss of Liver function, given its relationship to mental function and stress, may cause the mind to become active earlier in the morning than normal, thus awakening one.

Given that another of the Liver's 600 functions is to purify the bloodstream, reducing or eliminating the intake of toxic chemicals is very important as part of a larger strategy to resolve depression. It is also important to exercise vigorously (to a point of perspiration) for at least 30 minutes four times weekly, thus increasing Liver circulation, soothing the Liver and stimulating increased circulation throughout the body, which allows the body to detoxify at least to a small degree.

As you can see with this particular health problem, there is an underlying cause. The key to success in treating these problems lies in addressing the underlying issue described above to eliminate the

problem over the long term. To speed Acupuncture and/or Chinese Herbal Medicine results, it is recommended one minimally reduce or eliminate the intake of caffeine, deep-fried foods, dairy, sugar, preservatives in food, chemicals in food and municipal tap water (which most often contains chlorine and fluoride, considered by many as dangerous chemicals).

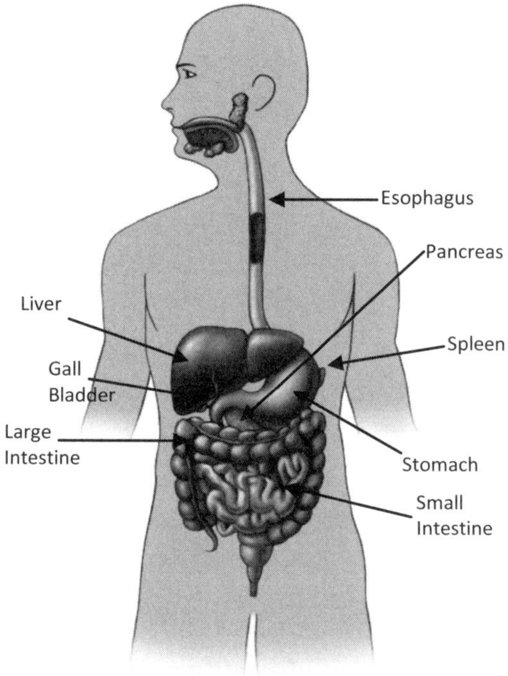

Menopausal Mood Swings

Menopausal mood swings have many potential causes, however what follows are the basic mechanics. Thousands of years ago, physicians in China began to explore the nature of human emotion and discovered a direct link between emotion and the organ system. Having helped many people resolve emotional imbalances over the years, we've found the following to be accurate from the point of view of the physical body (obviously many factors exist in life that may trigger bodily malfunction which, in turn, could then trigger an emotional response). What is described below is the relationship between the emotions and physical body.

The Liver has 600 physiological functions, one of which is to help the body adapt to the mental and emotional stresses of life. In other words, if one's Liver is functioning at a high level, stress entering one's life has no physical effect; however, if one's Liver isn't functioning well, stress can have a negative effect on the body.

Liver malfunction can cause a person to experience excessive or inappropriate mood swings, anger, irritability, frustration, impatience, and/or depression. For example, a person with multiple emotional stresses over many years may experience suppressed Liver function. Then, the loss of a loved one could cause Liver function to drop dramatically, and the person could then begin to experience mood swings. On the other hand, a well-functioning Liver will cause one to be emotionally even and generally happy.

Mood swings can be caused by a breakdown in Liver function, not simply an imbalance in brain chemistry (the typical Western Medical view of this particular condition). Ironically, addressing only the brain chemistry with medication often leads to further difficulty resolving the problem as shown here: if one takes a medication for the mood swings (which may be caused by a Liver imbalance) and that medication reduces Liver function (the Liver, in its capacity as a blood purifier, will attempt to eliminate the chemical from the body), it makes it more difficult to treat the mood swings. This explains why a person may take a medication their entire life.....and the mood swings never fully resolve!

Given that one of the Liver's 600 functions is to purify the bloodstream, reducing or eliminating the intake of toxic chemicals is very important as part of a larger strategy to resolve mood swings. It is also important to exercise vigorously (to a point of perspiration) for at least 30 minutes four times weekly, thus increasing Liver circulation, soothing the Liver and stimulating increased circulation throughout the body, which allows the body to detoxify at least to a small degree.

As you can see with this particular health problem, there is an underlying cause. The key to success in treating these problems lies in addressing the underlying issue described above to eliminate the problem over the long term. To speed Acupuncture and/or Chinese Herbal Medicine results, it is recommended one minimally reduce or eliminate the intake of caffeine, deep-fried foods, dairy, sugar, preservatives in food, chemicals in food and municipal tap water (which most often contains chlorine and fluoride, considered by many as dangerous chemicals).

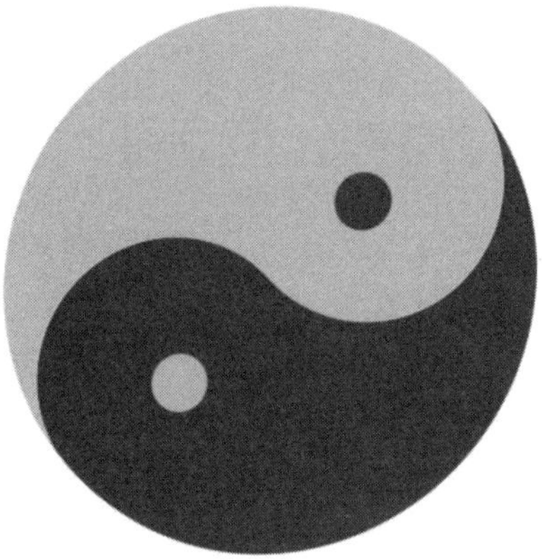

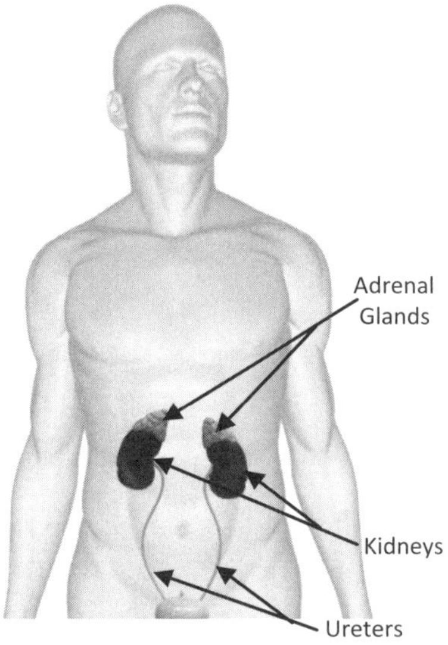

Menopausal Night Sweats

Menopausal night sweats have many potential causes, however what follows are the basic mechanics. Lack of Kidney/Adrenal system function can lead to inadequate raw materials necessary for the production of reproductive hormones, thus leading to night sweats. Two basic aspects of the Kidney/Adrenal system are "yin" and "yang." (See diagram above on the left.) Yin is cool, moist, and nourishing (an example of this would be the amniotic fluid around a baby in a woman's womb). On the other hand, yang is hot, invigorating and moving (an example of yang gone "awry" would be a woman experiencing night sweats). Female reproductive hormones have either more yin or more yang properties; for example, estrogen (which helps prepare the body for and maintain a pregnancy) may have more yang properties and progesterone (which helps prepare the uterus for receiving and nourishing a fertilized egg) may have more yin properties. Reproductive hormone balance (therefore Kidney yin and yang balance) is critical for normal body temperature.

When such hormones slip out of balance, many symptoms, including night sweats, may result. The yin may become deficient, causing the yang to “rise” to the surface of the body at night (the most yin time of day), causing an intense sensation of heat and possibly perspiration.

As you can see with this particular health problem, there is an underlying cause. The key to success in treating these problems lies in addressing the underlying issue described above to eliminate the problem over the long term. To speed Acupuncture and/or Chinese Herbal Medicine results, it is recommended one minimally reduce or eliminate the intake of caffeine, deep-fried foods, dairy, sugar, preservatives in food, chemicals in food and municipal tap water (which most often contains chlorine and fluoride, considered by many as dangerous chemicals).

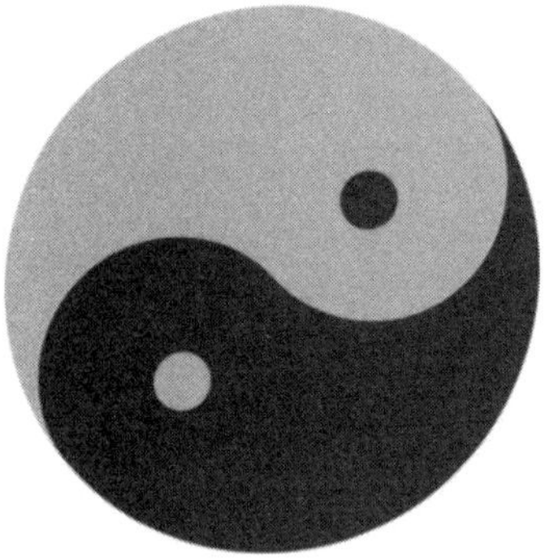

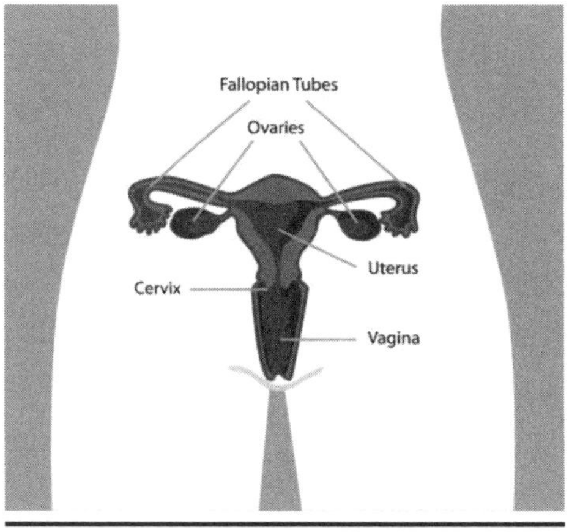

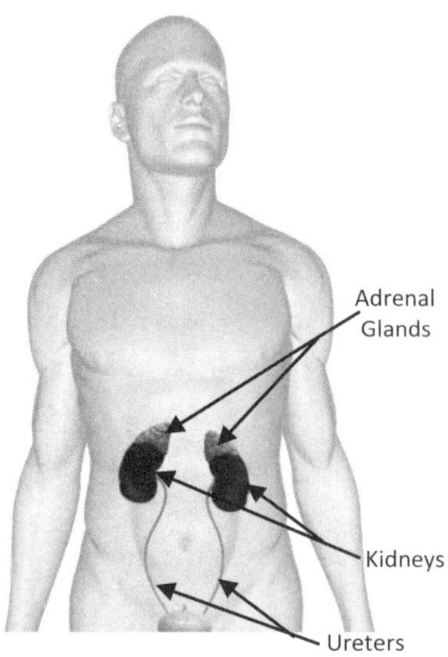

Menopausal Vaginal Dryness

Menopausal vaginal dryness has many potential causes, however what follows are the basic mechanics. Lack of Kidney/Adrenal system function can lead to inadequate raw materials necessary for the production of reproductive hormones, thus leading to vaginal dryness.

Two basic aspects of the Kidney/Adrenal system are "yin" and "yang." (See diagram above on far left.) Yin is cool, moist, and nourishing (an example of this is vaginal fluids). On the other hand, yang is hot, dry, invigorating and moving (an example of a lack of yang would be inadequate "digestive fire" causing weight gain). Female reproductive hormones have either more yin or more yang properties; for example, estrogen (which helps prepare the body for and maintain a pregnancy) may have more yang properties and progesterone (which helps prepare the uterus for receiving and nourishing a fertilized egg) may have more yin properties. Reproductive hormone balance (therefore Kidney yin and yang balance) is critical for normal tissue moisture.

When such hormones slip out of balance, many symptoms, including vaginal dryness, may result. When the yin is deficient, the yang can dry out the body's fluids, including vaginal fluids.

As you can see with this particular health problem, there is an underlying cause. The key to success in treating these problems lies in addressing the underlying issue described above to eliminate the problem over the long term. To speed Acupuncture and/or Chinese Herbal Medicine results, it is recommended one minimally reduce or eliminate the intake of caffeine, deep-fried foods, dairy, sugar, preservatives in food, chemicals in food and municipal tap water (which most often contains chlorine and fluoride, considered by many as dangerous chemicals).

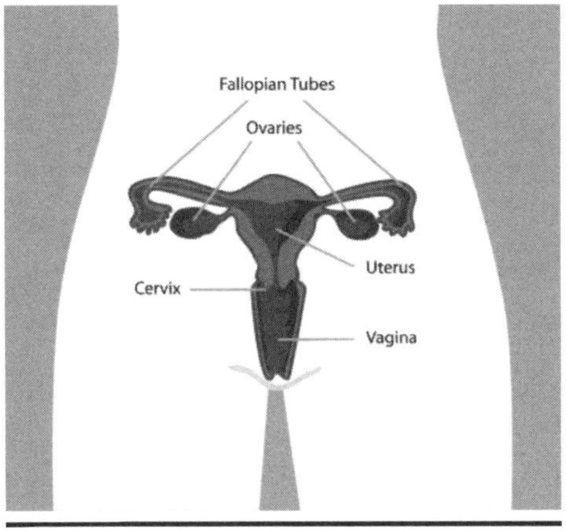

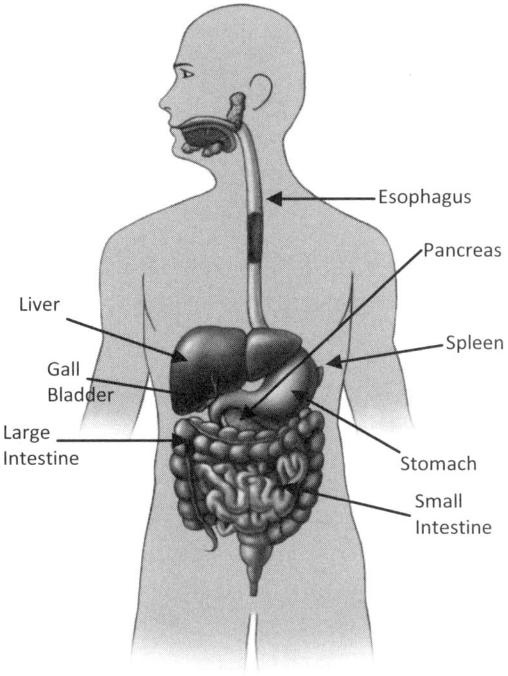

Menstrual Clotting

Menstrual clotting has many potential causes, however what follows are the basic mechanics. The Liver has 600 physiological functions, one of which is to encourage free blood and energy circulation throughout the body. Clots are simply the result of lost Liver function, causing blood to coagulate.

The following attributes illustrate high female reproductive system function:

- Timing: menstruation should coincide with the new moon and ovulation should occur during the full moon (if the moon phases can affect the oceans' tides, it can certainly affect body fluids)
- Duration: typically, flow should last 3-5 days
- Color: should be a healthy, red without abnormalities such as purple, pink, pale, brown, or black
- Amount: moderate at onset, a slight increase at midpoint, followed by a slight decrease just before ending (there should not be particularly heavy flow at any point)

- The rest of the month should pass without symptoms.

It can be very upsetting to some when they find out what a normal menstrual cycle should be. Do not take offense; the intention is to not upset, rather to simply outline a normal reproductive cycle. Thankfully, when one's menstrual cycle normalizes, menopause is a very smooth and effortless process that passes very quickly without significant abnormal symptoms.

Given that one of the Liver's 600 functions is to purify the bloodstream, reducing or eliminating the intake of toxic chemicals is very important as part of a larger strategy to resolve menstrual clotting. It is also important to exercise vigorously (to a point of perspiration) for at least 30 minutes four times weekly, thus increasing Liver circulation, soothing the Liver and stimulating increased circulation throughout the body, which allows the body to detoxify at least to a small degree.

As you can see with this particular health problem, there is an underlying cause. The key to success in treating these problems lies in addressing the underlying issue described above to eliminate the problem over the long term. To speed Acupuncture and/or Chinese Herbal Medicine results, it is recommended one minimally reduce or eliminate the intake of caffeine, deep-fried foods, dairy, sugar, preservatives in food, chemicals in food and municipal tap water (which most often contains chlorine and fluoride, considered by many as dangerous chemicals).

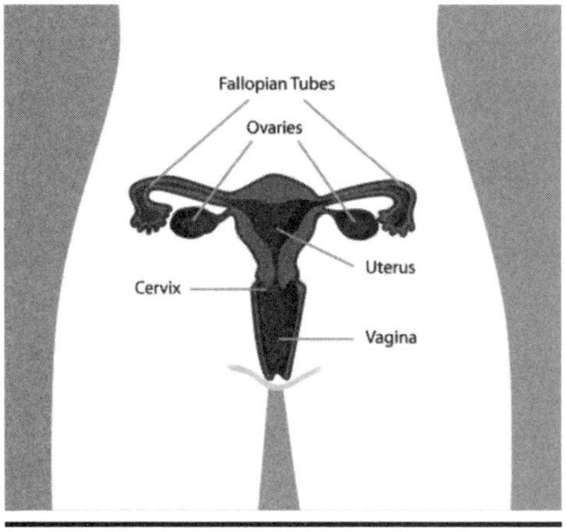

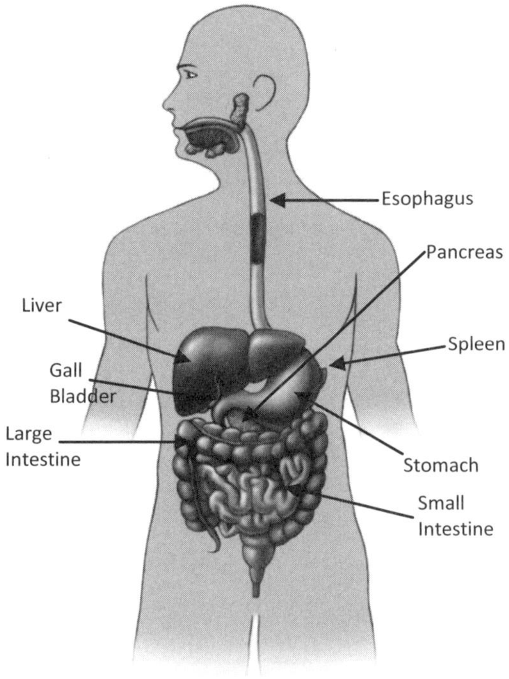

Menstrual Cramping

Cramping before or during menstruation has many potential causes, however what follows are the basic mechanics. The Liver has 600 physiological functions, one of which is to encourage free blood and energy circulation throughout the body. Cramping is simply the result of lost Liver function, causing circulation to stagnate, leading to pain.

The following attributes illustrate high female reproductive system function:

- Timing: menstruation should coincide with the new moon and ovulation should occur during the full moon (if the moon phases can affect the oceans' tides, it can certainly affect body fluids)
- Duration: typically, flow should last 3-5 days
- Color: should be healthy, red without abnormalities such as purple, pink, pale, brown, or black

- Amount: moderate at onset, a slight increase at midpoint, followed by a slight decrease just before ending (there should not be particularly heavy flow at any point)
- The rest of the month should pass without symptoms.

It can be very upsetting to some when they find out what a normal menstrual cycle should be. Do not take offense; the intention is to not upset, rather to simply outline a normal reproductive cycle. Thankfully, when one's menstrual cycle normalizes, menopause is a very smooth and effortless process that passes very quickly without significant abnormal symptoms.

Given that one of the Liver's 600 functions is to purify the bloodstream, reducing or eliminating the intake of toxic chemicals is very important as part of a larger strategy to resolve menstrual clotting. It is also important to exercise vigorously (to a point of perspiration) for at least 30 minutes four times weekly, thus increasing Liver circulation, soothing the Liver and stimulating increased circulation throughout the body, which allows the body to detoxify at least to a small degree.

As you can see with this particular health problem, there is an underlying cause. The key to success in treating these problems lies in addressing the underlying issue described above to eliminate the problem over the long term. To speed Acupuncture and/or Chinese Herbal Medicine results, it is recommended one minimally reduce or eliminate the intake of caffeine, deep-fried foods, dairy, sugar, preservatives in food, chemicals in food and municipal tap water (which most often contains chlorine and fluoride, considered by many as dangerous chemicals).

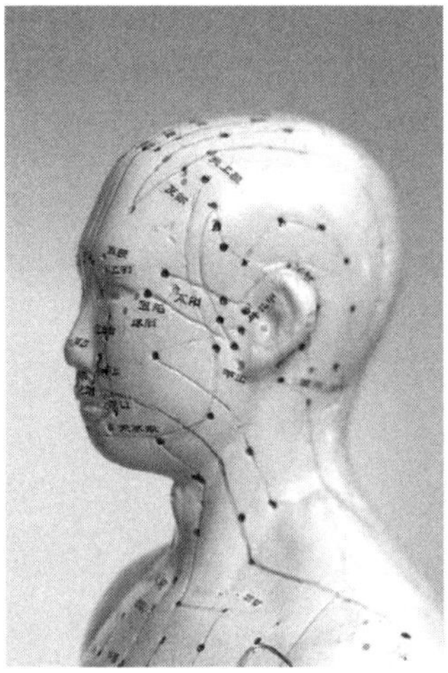

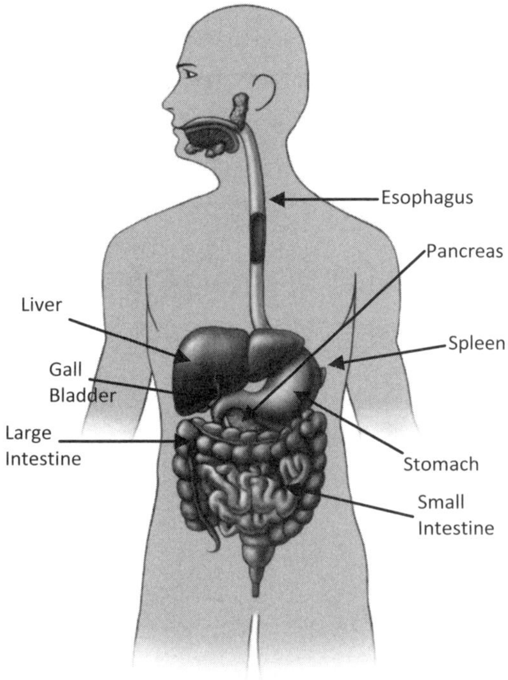

Migraines

Migraines have many potential causes, however what follows are the basic mechanics. Poor Liver and/or Gall Bladder function cause a significant number of migraines, as explained below.

The following illustrates the close relationship between the Liver and Gall Bladder as it relates to migraines: one of the Liver's 600 functions is to produce bile that is passed to the Gall Bladder and released into the intestine to "emulsify" (changing very large fat globules from food into much smaller fat droplets that can pass through the intestine wall and travel throughout the body in the bloodstream) fats upon consumption. The Liver also helps the body cope with life's emotional stresses and the Liver drives the blood and energy freely through the body in a relaxed fashion. In other words, if the Liver is functioning well, the blood vessels are relaxed and stable, whereas a loss of Liver function may lead to an inability to adapt to stress, resulting in blood vessel constriction, and finally Gall Bladder constriction, which may cause a referral of pain into the head, neck, and/or shoulders (see Gall Bladder connections to the head in the image above).

Migraines accompanied by eye and/or vision problems often indicate Liver involvement, as the Liver governs the functions of the eyes.

Digestive problems such as nausea that often accompany migraines may be caused by the Liver "overacting" on the digestive organs which, as you can see from the diagram above, are in very close proximity.

Given that another of the Liver's 600 functions is to purify the bloodstream, reducing or eliminating the intake of toxic chemicals is very important as part of a larger strategy to resolve migraines. It is also important to exercise vigorously (to a point of perspiration) for at least 30 minutes four times weekly, thus increasing Liver circulation, soothing the Liver and stimulating increased circulation throughout the body, which allows the body to detoxify at least to a small degree.

As you can see with this particular health problem, there is an underlying cause. The key to success in treating these problems lies in addressing the underlying issue described above to eliminate the problem over the long term. To speed Acupuncture and/or Chinese Herbal Medicine results, it is recommended one minimally reduce or eliminate the intake of caffeine, deep-fried foods, dairy, sugar, preservatives in food, chemicals in food and municipal tap water (which most often contains chlorine and fluoride, considered by many as dangerous chemicals).

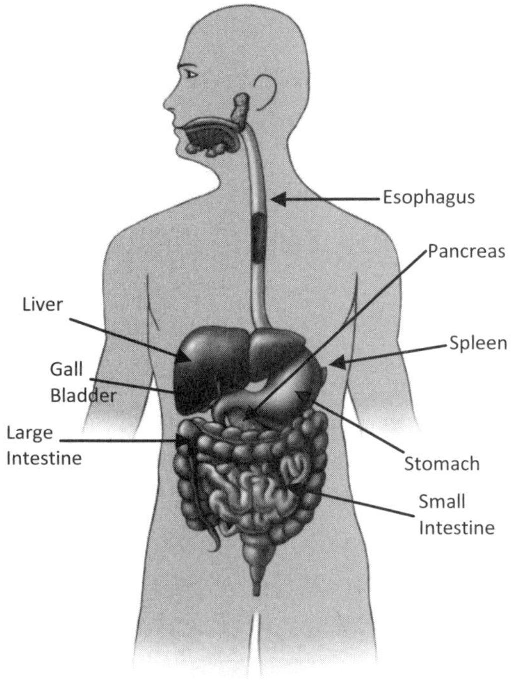

Mood Swings

Mood swings have many potential causes, however what follows are the basic mechanics. Thousands of years ago, physicians in China began to explore the nature of human emotion and discovered a direct link between emotion and the organ system. Having helped many people resolve emotional imbalances over the years, we've found the following to be accurate from the point of view of the physical body (obviously many factors exist in life that may trigger bodily malfunction which, in turn, could then trigger an emotional response). What is described below is the relationship between the emotions and physical body.

The Liver has 600 physiological functions, one of which is to help the body adapt to the mental and emotional stresses of life. In other words, if one's Liver is functioning at a high level, stress entering one's life has no physical effect; however, if one's Liver isn't functioning well, stress can have a negative effect on the body.

Liver malfunction can cause a person to experience excessive or inappropriate mood swings, anger, irritability, frustration, impatience, and/or depression. For example, a person with multiple emotional stresses over many years may experience suppressed Liver function. Then, the loss of a loved one could cause Liver function to drop dramatically, and the person could then begin to experience mood swings. On the other hand, a well-functioning Liver will cause one to be emotionally even and generally happy.

Mood swings can be caused by a breakdown in Liver function, not simply an imbalance in brain chemistry (the typical Western Medical view of this particular condition). Ironically, addressing only the brain chemistry with medication often leads to further difficulty resolving the problem as shown here: if one takes a medication for the mood swings (which may be caused by a Liver imbalance) and that medication reduces Liver function (the Liver, in its capacity as a blood purifier, will attempt to eliminate the chemical from the body), it makes it more difficult to treat the mood swings. This explains why a person may take a medication their entire life.....and the mood swings never fully resolve!

Given that one of the Liver's 600 functions is to purify the bloodstream, reducing or eliminating the intake of toxic chemicals is very important as part of a larger strategy to resolve mood swings. It is also important to exercise vigorously (to a point of perspiration) for at least 30 minutes four times weekly, thus increasing Liver circulation, soothing the Liver and stimulating increased circulation throughout the body, which allows the body to detoxify at least to a small degree.

As you can see with this particular health problem, there is an underlying cause. The key to success in treating these problems lies in addressing the underlying issue described above to eliminate the problem over the long term. To speed Acupuncture and/or Chinese Herbal Medicine results, it is recommended one minimally reduce or eliminate the intake of caffeine, deep-fried foods, dairy, sugar, preservatives in food, chemicals in food and municipal tap water (which most often contains chlorine and fluoride, considered by many as dangerous chemicals).

Muscle Cramping

Muscle cramping has many potential causes, however what follows are the basic mechanics. Every muscle in the body requires adequate blood flow which delivers the nutrients necessary for its function, such as potassium, calcium, etc.

Muscle cramping is caused by a lack of blood circulation or any combination of its constituents to the affected area; muscle cramping is resolved by restoring normal blood circulation to the area involved.

As you can see with this particular health problem, there is an underlying cause. The key to success in treating these problems lies in addressing the underlying issue described above to eliminate the problem over the long term. To speed Acupuncture and/or Chinese Herbal Medicine results, it is recommended one drink adequate water, use electrolytes and minimally reduce or eliminate the intake of caffeine, deep-fried foods, dairy, sugar, preservatives in food, chemicals in food and municipal tap water (which most often contains chlorine and fluoride, considered by many as dangerous chemicals).

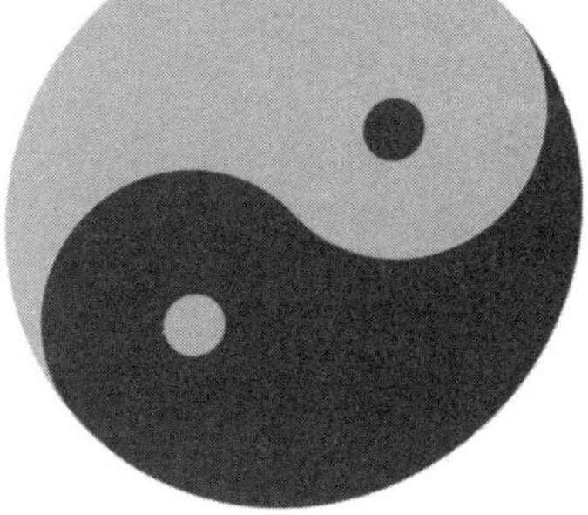

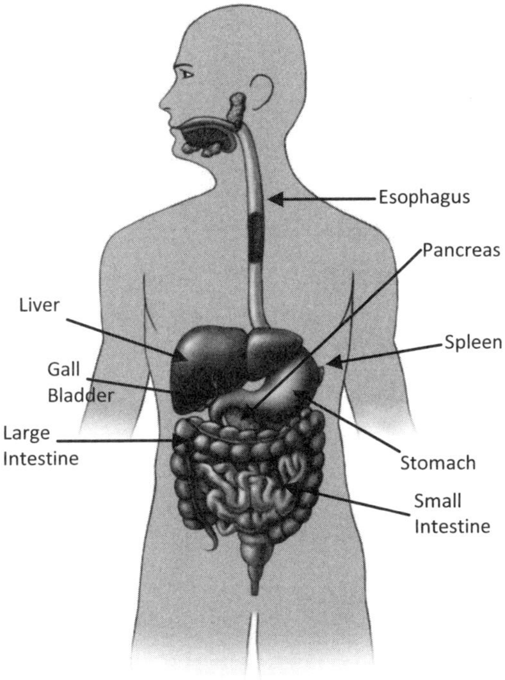

Narcolepsy

Narcolepsy has many potential causes, however what follows are the basic mechanics.

1. The Stomach and Spleen/Pancreatic system are responsible for a certain amount of energy production, which begins with nutrients being extracted from food in the Stomach, in part due to the actions of the Spleen/Pancreatic system. Those nutrients are then sent into the intestines, pass through the intestine wall into the blood stream and travel throughout the body, stimulating processes that give one energy. Regardless of how well one eats, lack of Stomach and/or Spleen/Pancreatic system function may lead to an uncontrollable desire to fall asleep.

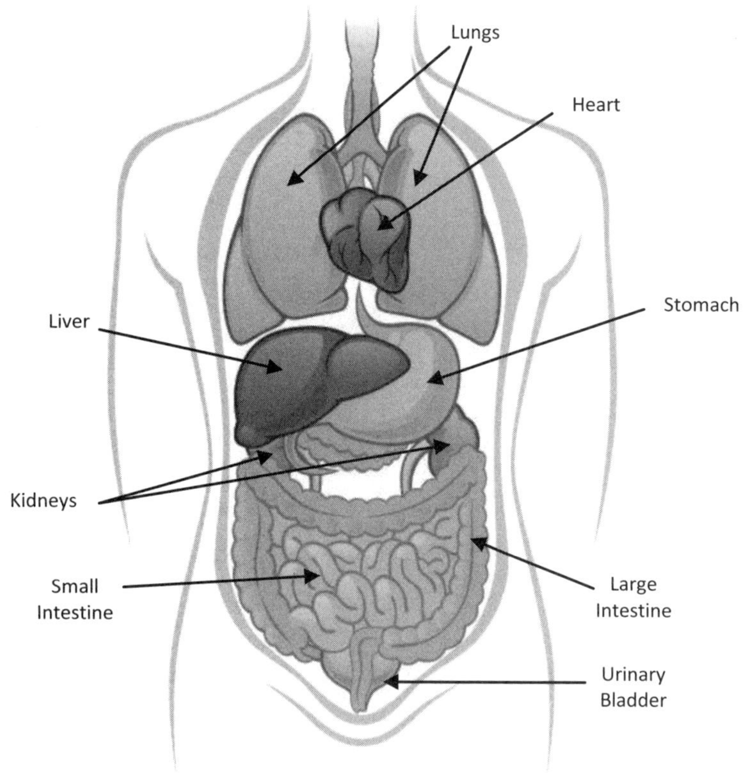

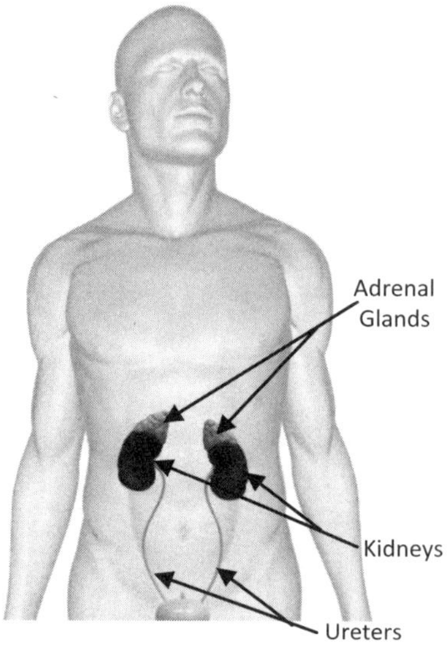

2. The Lungs bring oxygen into the body, which then travels in the bloodstream to the brain giving one energy. Lack of Lung function may cause an uncontrollable desire to fall asleep.

3. Kidney/Adrenal system weakness may also cause an uncontrollable desire to fall asleep. The Kidney/Adrenal system produces raw materials for the production of hormones (for example, testosterone) the body uses to control many functions including energy production; the Kidney/Adrenal system also produces and releases adrenaline, and may become depleted by long-term inadequate sleep, excessive mental stress and/or excessive physical stress. Two basic aspects of the Kidney/Adrenal system are "yin" and "yang." The yin is cool, moist, and nourishing (an example of this would be like the amniotic fluid around a baby). On the other hand, yang is hot, invigorating and moving (an example of yang is the force necessary to keep one's eyelids open). All of

the body's hormones have either more yin or more yang properties for example, testosterone has very yang properties that are vital to drive energy levels. Narcolepsy can be caused by a "yang deficiency," leading to difficulty keeping one's eyes open in the daytime.

As you can see with this particular health problem, there is an underlying cause. The key to success in treating these problems lies in addressing the underlying issue described above to eliminate the problem over the long term. To speed Acupuncture and/or Chinese Herbal Medicine results, it is recommended one increase protein in ratio to carbohydrates at every meal and minimally reduce or eliminate the intake of caffeine, deep-fried foods, dairy, sugar, preservatives in food, chemicals in food and municipal tap water (which most often contains chlorine and fluoride, considered by many as dangerous chemicals).

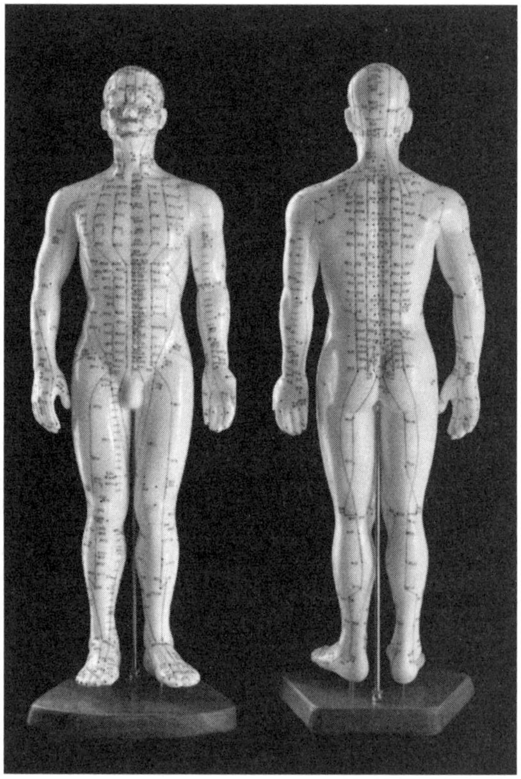

Neuropathy: Finger, Hand, Arm, Toe, Foot, Leg

Neuropathy has many potential causes, however what follows are the basic possibilities (Diabetes is one potential complicating factor in any of the cases below):

1. Nerve damage in any part of the body may often cause a person to experience strange, shooting pains.

2. A loss of blood circulation in any part of the body may cause a sensation of numbness.

3. Reduced energy circulation may cause dull pain.

4. Severe lack of blood flow and/or scar tissue (see section "Pain due to Scar Tissue") may cause sharp pain.

Any or all of the above may be involved when one experiences neuropathy.

As you can see with this particular health problem, there is an underlying cause. The key to success in treating these problems lies in addressing the underlying issue described above to eliminate the problem over the long term. To speed Acupuncture and/or Chinese Herbal Medicine results, it is recommended one increase protein in ratio to carbohydrates at every meal and minimally reduce or eliminate the intake of caffeine, deep-fried foods, dairy, sugar, preservatives in food, chemicals in food and municipal tap water (which most often contains chlorine and fluoride, considered by many as dangerous chemicals).

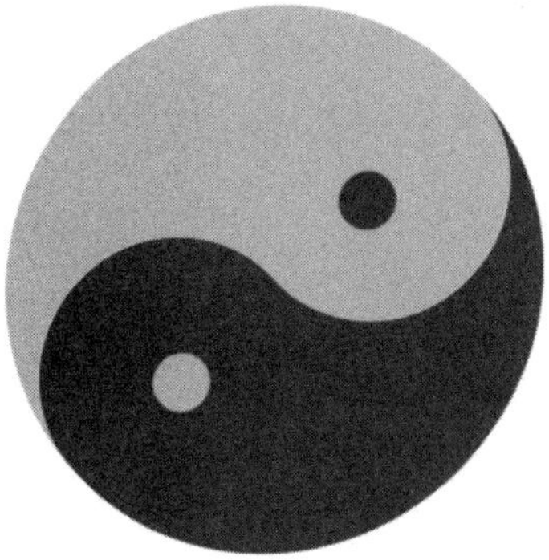

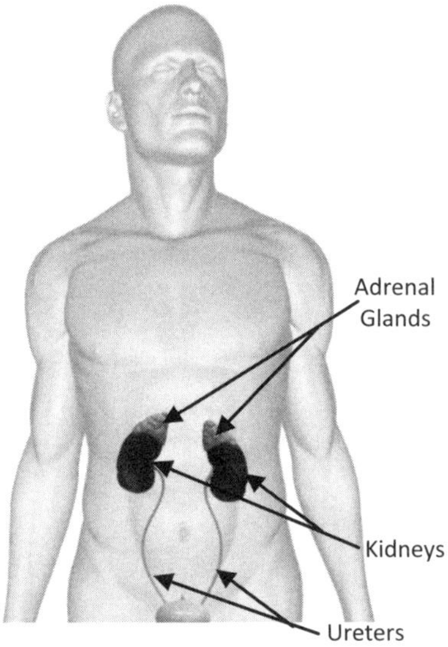

Night Sweats/ Excessive Heat at Night

Night sweats have many potential causes, however what follows are the basic mechanics. Lack of Kidney/Adrenal system function can lead to inadequate raw materials necessary for the production of hormones, thus leading to night sweats. Two basic aspects of the Kidney/Adrenal system are "yin" and "yang." (See diagram above on the left.) Yin is cool, moist, and nourishing (an example of this would be the amniotic fluid around a baby in a woman's womb). On the other hand, yang is hot, invigorating and moving (an example of yang gone "awry" would be one experiencing night sweats). Hormones have either more yin or more yang properties for example, estrogen (which helps prepare the body for and maintain a pregnancy) may have more yang properties and progesterone (which helps prepare the uterus for receiving and nourishing a fertilized egg) may have more yin properties. Hormone balance (therefore Kidney yin and yang balance) is critical for normal body temperature.

When such hormones slip out of balance, many symptoms, including night sweats, may result. The yin may become deficient, causing the yang to “rise” to the surface of the body at night (the most yin time of day), causing an intense sensation of heat and possibly perspiration.

As you can see with this particular health problem, there is an underlying cause. The key to success in treating these problems lies in addressing the underlying issue described above to eliminate the problem over the long term. To speed Acupuncture and/or Chinese Herbal Medicine results, it is recommended one minimally reduce or eliminate the intake of caffeine, deep-fried foods, dairy, sugar, preservatives in food, chemicals in food and municipal tap water (which most often contains chlorine and fluoride, considered by many as dangerous chemicals).

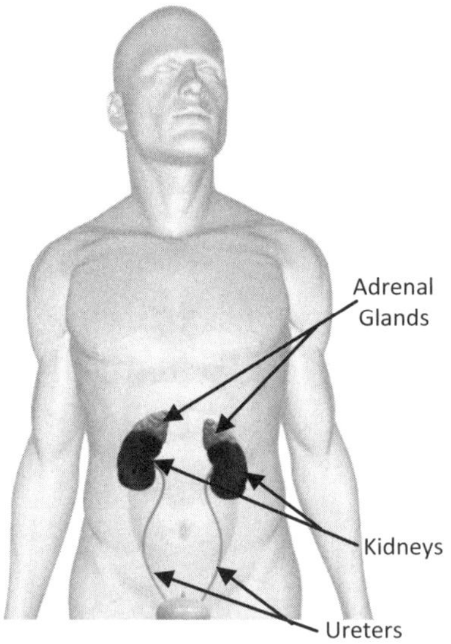

Osteoporosis

Osteoporosis has many potential causes, however what follows are the basic mechanics. Osteoporosis is most often caused by a loss of Kidney/Adrenal system function; the Kidney/Adrenal system produces raw materials for many hormones that drive bodily functions, including "osteoblasts" (cells that build bone tissue) and "osteoclasts" (cells that break down bone tissue). Abnormal Kidney/Adrenal system function may lead to abnormal ratios of these hormones, causing bone tissue problems such as osteoporosis.

As you can see with this particular health problem, there is an underlying cause. The key to success in treating these problems lies in addressing the underlying issue described above to eliminate the problem over the long term. To speed Acupuncture and/or Chinese Herbal Medicine results, it is recommended one minimally reduce or eliminate the intake of caffeine, deep-fried foods, dairy, sugar, preservatives in food, chemicals in food and municipal tap water (which most often contains chlorine and fluoride, considered by many as dangerous chemicals).

Pain Due to Scar Tissue

Pain due to scar tissue can be very uncomfortable and last for years if left untreated; what follows are the basic mechanics. To understand this type of pain, one must understand that muscle tissue has a "grain" similar to that of wood. Physical trauma can tear the muscle tissue and, upon healing, dead and fibrous material (scar tissue) may fill the space between the very fine muscle fibers. If the tear is small, the body has a chance of healing that area. If the tear is large and the body is not capable of reconnecting the tissue, web-like tissue without circulation may settle in the area, blocking circulation and leading to pain.

One reason scar tissue may exist in the human body post-trauma lies in the fact that it seems in many cases there is not adequate energy required for large muscle repairs. Most energy in the human body is used for brain function and mental capacity (as compared to the relatively small amount of energy used by the body for physical activity); many animals (as an example, salamanders, amazingly, can regenerate lost limbs....although they have very little, if any, cognitive function) have more evenly distributed energy.

Using Acupuncture, the first step is encouraging the energy and blood to re-route around the scar tissue to reduce the pain and discomfort. Then, in order to dissolve the scar tissue, Acupuncture drives circulation (bringing nutrients, hormones and oxygen) into the area that may dissolve scar tissue. Eventually, torn muscle fibers may reconnect, thus reinstating normal circulation and eliminating the source of the pain.

As you can see with this particular health problem, there is an underlying cause. The key to success in treating these problems lies in addressing the underlying issue described above to eliminate the problem over the long term. To speed Acupuncture and/or Chinese Herbal Medicine results, it is recommended one minimally reduce or eliminate the intake of caffeine, deep-fried foods, dairy, sugar, preservatives in food, chemicals in food and municipal tap water (which most often contains chlorine and fluoride, considered by many as dangerous chemicals).

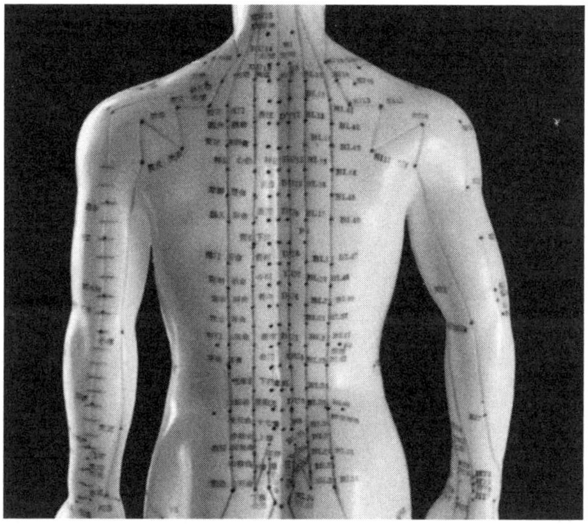

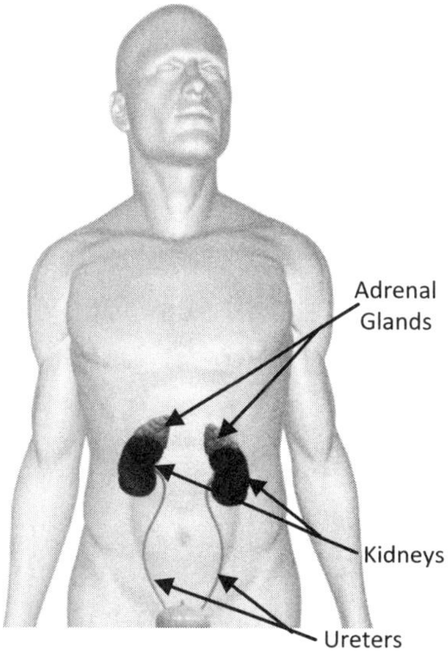

Pain: Lower Back

Lower back pain has many potential causes, however what follows are basic possibilities:

1. Trauma or injury can cause a problem with blood, nerve, and/or energy circulation in the lower back. Scar tissue may result, complicating the condition (see section "Pain due to Scar Tissue").

2. Kidney/Adrenal system governs the function and structure of the lower back. If the Kidney/Adrenal system function declines, they may shrink (perhaps as little as several millimeters) causing the surrounding muscle tissue to fill the resulting space. Such muscle changes may, in turn, cut off circulation and/or pull the spine's vertebral bones out of place, causing an impingement of the nerve and pain. Nerve damage in any part of the body may often cause a person to experience strange, shooting pains.

3. Reduced energy circulation may cause dull pain.

4. Severe lack of blood circulation and/or scar tissue (see section "Pain due to Scar Tissue") may cause sharp pain.

Any or all of the above may be involved when one experiences lower back pain.

As you can see with this particular health problem, there is an underlying cause. The key to success in treating these problems lies in addressing the underlying issue described above to eliminate the problem over the long term. To speed Acupuncture and/or Chinese Herbal Medicine results, it is recommended one minimally reduce or eliminate the intake of caffeine, deep-fried foods, dairy, sugar, preservatives in food, chemicals in food and municipal tap water (which most often contains chlorine and fluoride, considered by many as dangerous chemicals).

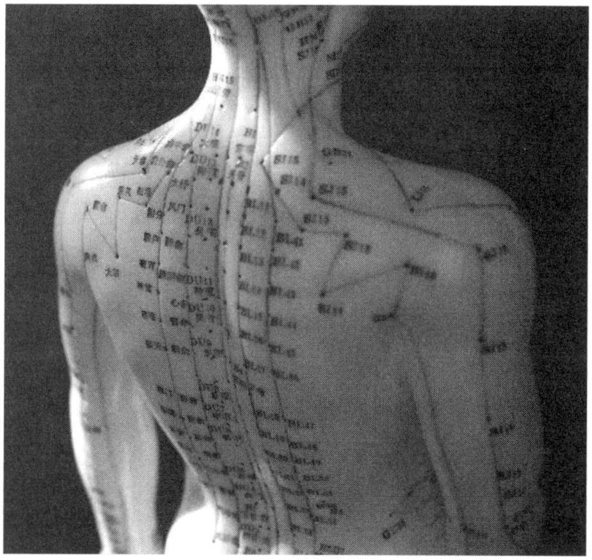

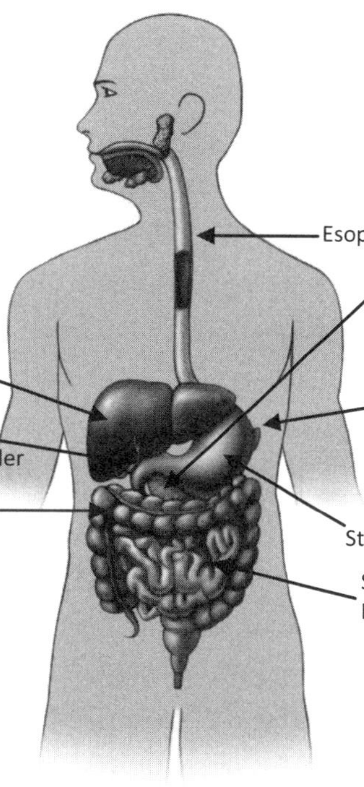

Pain: Neck, Arm, Shoulder and Elbow

Pain in the neck, arm, shoulder and/or elbow regions has many potential causes, however what follows are the basic mechanics. The exact location of the pain is one of the more important parts of diagnosing the cause of the pain in this part of the body. For example, if the pain was on a specific pathway, it may be related to that specific organ (see diagrams above).

For example, the Liver has 600 physiological functions, including being responsible for helping the body deal with the mental and emotional stresses and traumas of life. Over time with long-term stress, the Liver can break down and cause problems for the Gall Bladder. The Gall Bladder will then refer pain to the neck or shoulder region on that specific pathway, where decreased energy circulation may cause dull pain, whereas impaired blood circulation and/or scar tissue (see section "Pain due to Scar Tissue") may cause sharp pain.

Nerve damage in any part of the body may often cause a person to experience strange, shooting pains.

Any or all of the above may be involved when one experiences pain in those areas.

As you can see with this particular health problem, there is an underlying cause. The key to success in treating these problems lies in addressing the underlying issue described above to eliminate the problem over the long term. To speed Acupuncture and/or Chinese Herbal Medicine results, it is recommended one minimally reduce or eliminate the intake of caffeine, deep-fried foods, dairy, sugar, preservatives in food, chemicals in food and municipal tap water (which most often contains chlorine and fluoride, considered by many as dangerous chemicals).

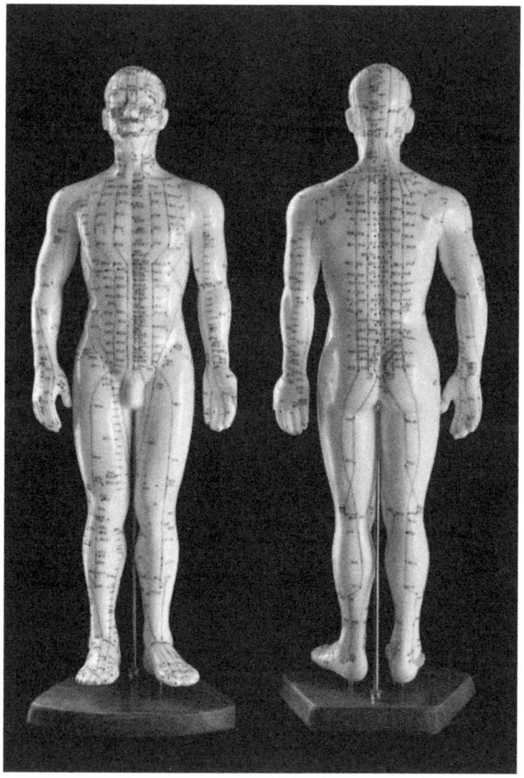

Pain: Upper Back, Lower Back, Arm, Leg, and Joints

Pain in the body has many potential causes, however what follows are the basic possibilities:

1. Nerve damage in any part of the body may often cause a person to experience strange, shooting pains.

2. A loss of blood circulation in any part of the body may cause a sensation of numbness.

3. Reduced energy circulation may cause dull pain.

4. Severe lack of blood circulation and/or scar tissue (see section "Pain due to Scar Tissue") may cause sharp pain.

Any or all of the above may be involved when one experiences pain.

As you can see with this particular health problem, there is an underlying cause. The key to success in treating these problems lies in addressing the underlying issue described above to eliminate the problem over the long term. To speed Acupuncture and/or Chinese Herbal Medicine results, it is recommended one increase protein in ratio to carbohydrates at every meal and minimally reduce or eliminate the intake of caffeine, deep-fried foods, dairy, sugar, preservatives in food, chemicals in food and municipal tap water (which most often contains chlorine and fluoride, considered by many as dangerous chemicals).

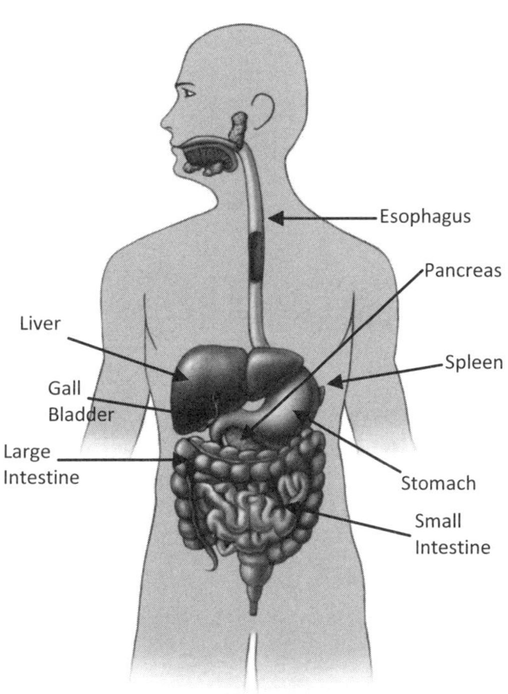

Parkinson's Disease

Parkinson's disease has many potential causes, however what follows are three possible causes, one or all of which may be involved:

1. Every muscle in the body requires a certain amount of blood circulation, delivering hormones, oxygen and nutrients such as potassium, calcium, etc. to the affected area. Muscles in the affected area may not receive adequate blood circulation, leading to involuntary movement.

2. Nervous system malfunction can cause abnormal muscle movement.

3. Liver malfunction may lead to abnormal muscle movement.

Given that one of the Liver's 600 functions is to purify the bloodstream, reducing or eliminating the intake of toxic chemicals is very important as part of a larger strategy to alleviating Parkinson's. It is also important to exercise vigorously (if possible and with your doctor's supervision) to a point of perspiration for at least 30 minutes four times weekly, thus increasing Liver circulation, soothing the Liver and stimulating increased circulation throughout the body, which allows the body to detoxify at least to a small degree.

As you can see with this particular health problem, there is an underlying cause. The key to success in treating these problems lies in addressing the underlying issue described above to eliminate the problem over the long term. To speed Acupuncture and/or Chinese Herbal Medicine results, it is recommended one minimally reduce or eliminate the intake of caffeine, deep-fried foods, dairy, sugar, preservatives in food, chemicals in food and municipal tap water (which most often contains chlorine and fluoride, considered by many as dangerous chemicals).

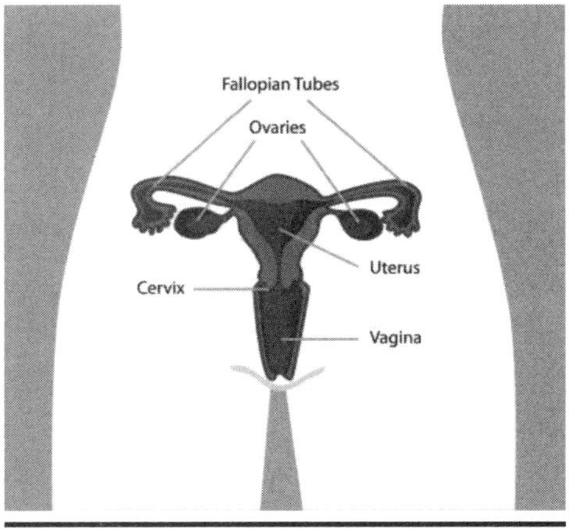

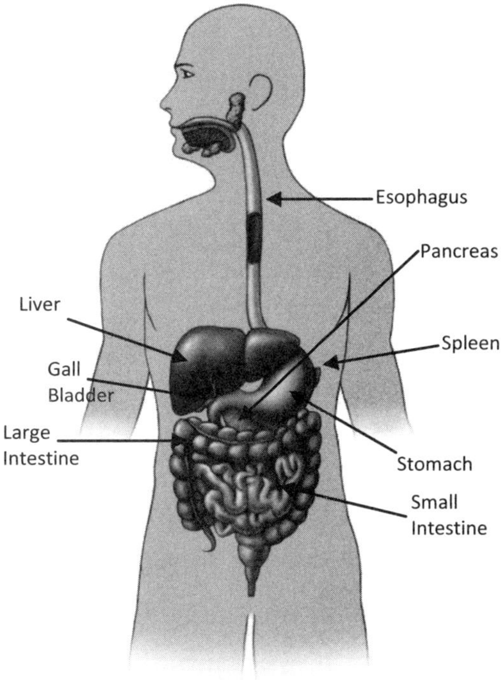

Pre-Menstrual Cramping

Cramping before and/or during menstruation has many potential causes, however what follows are the basic mechanics. The Liver has 600 physiological functions, one of which is to encourage free blood and energy circulation throughout the body. Cramping is simply the result of lost Liver function, causing circulation to stagnate, leading to pain.

The following attributes illustrate high female reproductive system function:

- Timing: menstruation should coincide with the new moon and ovulation should occur during the full moon (if the moon phases can affect the oceans' tides, it can certainly affect body fluids)
- Duration: typically, flow should last 3-5 days
- Color: should be healthy, red without abnormalities such as purple, pink, pale, brown, or black

- Amount: moderate at onset, a slight increase at midpoint, followed by a slight decrease just before ending (there should not be particularly heavy flow at any point)
- The rest of the month should pass without symptoms.

It can be very upsetting to some when they find out what a normal menstrual cycle should be. Do not take offense; the intention is to not upset, rather to simply outline a normal reproductive cycle. Thankfully, when one's menstrual cycle normalizes, menopause is a very smooth and effortless process that passes very quickly without significant abnormal symptoms.

Given that one of the Liver's 600 functions is to purify the bloodstream, reducing or eliminating the intake of toxic chemicals is very important as part of a larger strategy to resolve pre-menstrual cramping. It is also important to exercise vigorously (to a point of perspiration) for at least 30 minutes four times weekly, thus increasing Liver circulation, soothing the Liver and stimulating increased circulation throughout the body, which allows the body to detoxify at least to a small degree.

As you can see with this particular health problem, there is an underlying cause. The key to success in treating these problems lies in addressing the underlying issue described above to eliminate the problem over the long term. To speed Acupuncture and/or Chinese Herbal Medicine results, it is recommended one minimally reduce or eliminate the intake of caffeine, deep-fried foods, dairy, sugar, preservatives in food, chemicals in food and municipal tap water (which most often contains chlorine and fluoride, considered by many as dangerous chemicals).

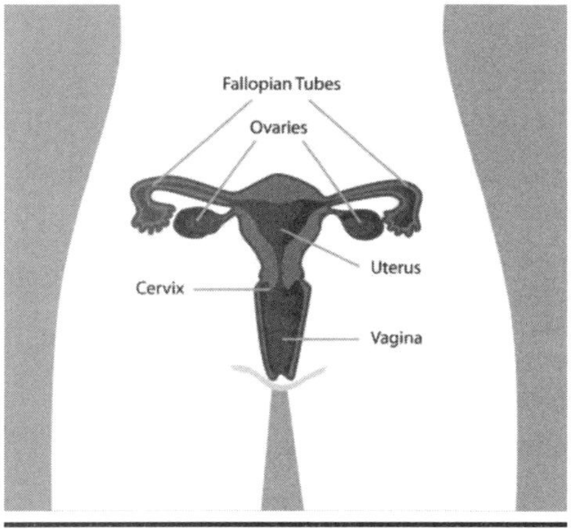

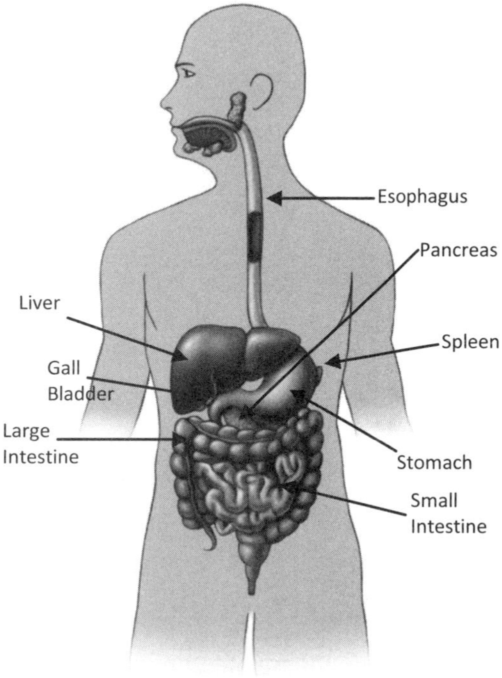

Pre-Menstrual Digestive problems

Pre-menstrual digestive problems take many forms and have many potential causes, however what follows are the basic mechanics. The Stomach receives the food and fluids one consumes via the esophagus and the Spleen/Pancreatic system (which also manufactures insulin, produces certain immune system cells) breaks down that food and fluid into usable nutrients that are sent to the intestines where they travel into the bloodstream through the intestine wall. The Liver produces bile which the Gall Bladder releases into the intestines to dissolve fats that you consume. The Small Intestine separates usable parts of food and fluids from the unusable, distributes the usable components throughout the body and eliminates the unusable components. Finally, the Large Intestine eliminates solid waste from the body.

If any one or more of the above systems are malfunctioning, it is vital to reinstate normal function to the affected area to resolve the digestive problems.

The following attributes illustrate high female reproductive system function:

- Timing: menstruation should coincide with the new moon and ovulation should occur during the full moon (if the moon phases can affect the oceans' tides, it can certainly affect body fluids)
- Duration: typically, flow should last 3-5 days
- Color: should be healthy, red without abnormalities such as purple, pink, pale, brown, or black
- Amount: moderate at onset, a slight increase at midpoint, followed by a slight decrease just before ending (there should not be particularly heavy flow at any point)
- The rest of the month, including the days leading up to menstruation, should pass without symptoms, digestive or otherwise.

It can be very upsetting to some when they find out what a normal menstrual cycle should be. Do not take offense; the intention is to not upset, rather to simply outline a normal reproductive cycle. Thankfully, when one's menstrual cycle normalizes, menopause is a very smooth and effortless process that passes very quickly without significant abnormal symptoms.

Given that one of the Liver's 600 functions is to purify the bloodstream, reducing or eliminating the intake of toxic chemicals is very important as part of a larger strategy to resolve digestive problems. It is also important to exercise vigorously (to a point of perspiration) for at least 30 minutes four times weekly, thus increasing Liver circulation, soothing the Liver and stimulating increased circulation throughout the body, which allows the body to detoxify at least to a small degree.

As you can see with this particular health problem, there is an underlying cause. The key to success in treating these problems lies in addressing the underlying issue described above to eliminate the

problem over the long term. To speed Acupuncture and/or Chinese Herbal Medicine results, it is recommended one minimally reduce or eliminate the intake of caffeine, deep-fried foods, dairy, sugar, preservatives in food, chemicals in food and municipal tap water (which most often contains chlorine and fluoride, considered by many as dangerous chemicals).

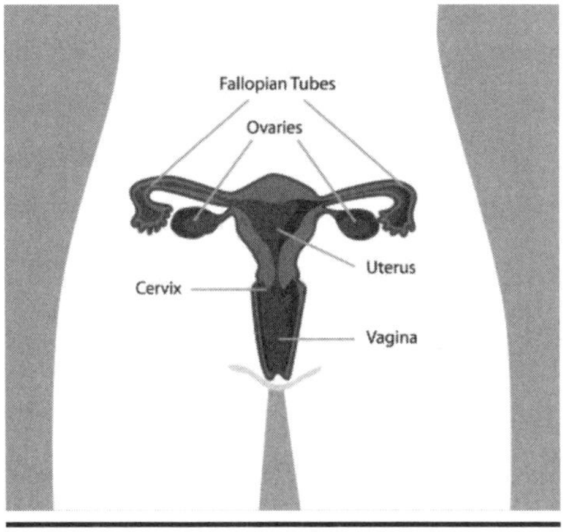

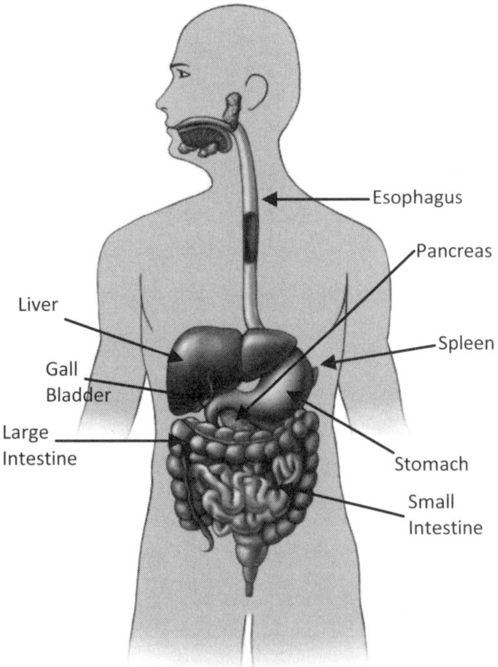

Pre-Menstrual Mood Swings

Pre-menstrual mood swings have many potential causes, however what follows are the basic mechanics. Thousands of years ago, physicians in China began to explore the nature of human emotion and discovered a direct link between emotion and the organ system. Having helped many people resolve emotional imbalances over the years, we've found the following to be accurate from the point of view of the physical body (obviously many factors exist in life that may trigger bodily malfunction which, in turn, could then trigger an emotional response). What is described below is the relationship between the emotions and physical body.

The Liver has 600 physiological functions, one of which is to help the body adapt to the mental and emotional stresses of life. In other words, if one's Liver is functioning at a high level, stress entering one's life has no physical effect; however, if one's Liver isn't functioning well, stress can have a negative effect on the body.

Liver malfunction can cause a person to experience excessive or inappropriate mood swings, anger, irritability, frustration, impatience, and/or depression. For example, a person with multiple emotional stresses over many years may experience suppressed Liver function. Then, the loss of a loved one could cause Liver function to drop dramatically, and the person could then begin to experience mood swings before menstruation. On the other hand, a well-functioning Liver will cause one to be emotionally even and generally happy.

Mood swings can be caused by a breakdown in Liver function, not simply an imbalance in brain chemistry (the typical Western Medical view of this particular condition). Ironically, addressing only the brain chemistry with medication often leads to further difficulty resolving the problem as shown here: if one takes a medication for the mood swings (which may be caused by a Liver imbalance) and that medication reduces Liver function (the Liver, in its capacity as a blood purifier, will attempt to eliminate the chemical from the body), it makes it more difficult to treat the mood swings. This explains why a person may take a medication their entire life.....and the mood swings never fully resolve!

Given that one of the Liver's 600 functions is to purify the bloodstream, reducing or eliminating the intake of toxic chemicals is very important as part of a larger strategy to resolve pre-menstrual mood swings. It is also important to exercise vigorously (to a point of perspiration) for at least 30 minutes four times weekly, thus increasing Liver circulation, soothing the Liver and stimulating increased circulation throughout the body, which allows the body to detoxify at least to a small degree.

The following attributes illustrate high female reproductive system function:

- Timing: menstruation should coincide with the new moon and ovulation should occur during the full moon (if the moon phases can affect the oceans' tides, it can certainly affect body fluids)
- Duration: typically, flow should last 3-5 days
- Color: should be healthy, red without abnormalities such as purple, pink, pale, brown, or black
- Amount: moderate at onset, a slight increase at midpoint, followed by a slight decrease just before ending (there should not be particularly heavy flow at any point)
- The rest of the month, including the days leading up to menstruation, should pass without symptoms, emotional or otherwise.

It can be very upsetting to some when they find out what a normal menstrual cycle should be. Do not take offense; the intention is to not upset, rather to simply outline a normal reproductive cycle. Thankfully, when one's menstrual cycle normalizes, menopause is a very smooth and effortless process that passes very quickly without significant abnormal symptoms.

As you can see with this particular health problem, there is an underlying cause. The key to success in treating these problems lies in addressing the underlying issue described above to eliminate the problem over the long term. To speed Acupuncture and/or Chinese Herbal Medicine results, it is recommended one minimally reduce or eliminate the intake of caffeine, deep-fried foods, dairy, sugar, preservatives in food, chemicals in food and municipal tap water (which most often contains chlorine and fluoride, considered by many as dangerous chemicals).

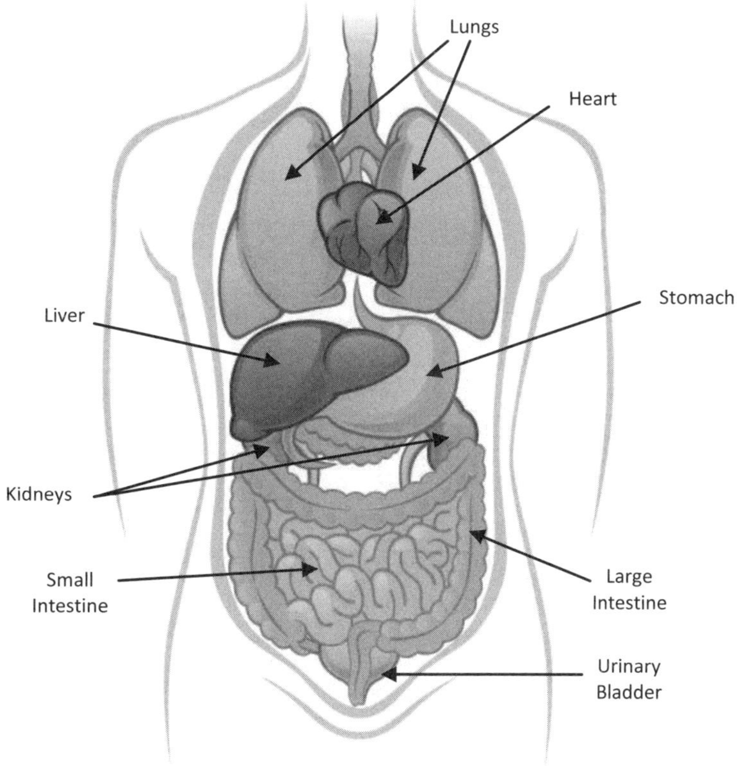

Post-Stroke Syndrome

A stroke and subsequent symptoms have many potential causes, however what follows are the basic mechanics. The Liver has 600 physiological functions, including helping the body adapt to the mental and emotional stresses of life, nourishing Heart function and encouraging adequate circulation throughout the body.

The stroke itself may be caused by long-term stress that decreases Liver function, leading to a breakdown in Heart function, which may lead to a blood clot that may break free and cause havoc. The subsequent loss of circulation may damage nerve tissue, leading to numbness, a lack of muscle function, a loss of nerve function, a loss of speech abilities and/or other unfortunate phenomena.

Given that one of the Liver's 600 functions is to purify the bloodstream, reducing or eliminating the intake of toxic chemicals is very important as part of a larger strategy to alleviate the symptoms related to a stroke.

As you can see with this particular health problem, there is an underlying cause. The key to success in treating these problems lies in addressing the underlying issue described above to eliminate the problem over the long term. To speed Acupuncture and/or Chinese Herbal Medicine results, it is recommended one minimally reduce or eliminate the intake of caffeine, deep-fried foods, dairy, sugar, preservatives in food, chemicals in food and municipal tap water (which most often contains chlorine and fluoride, considered by many as dangerous chemicals).

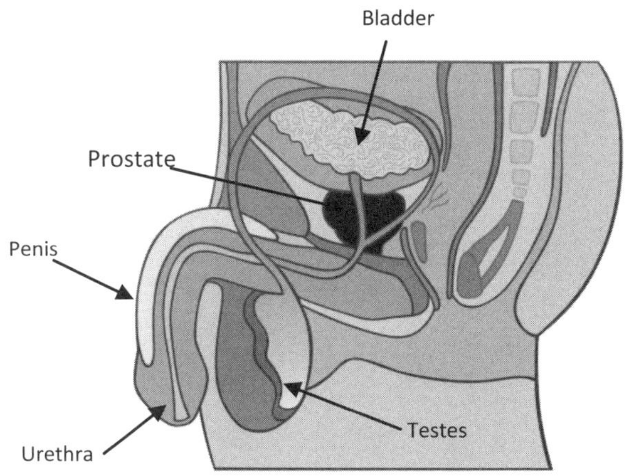

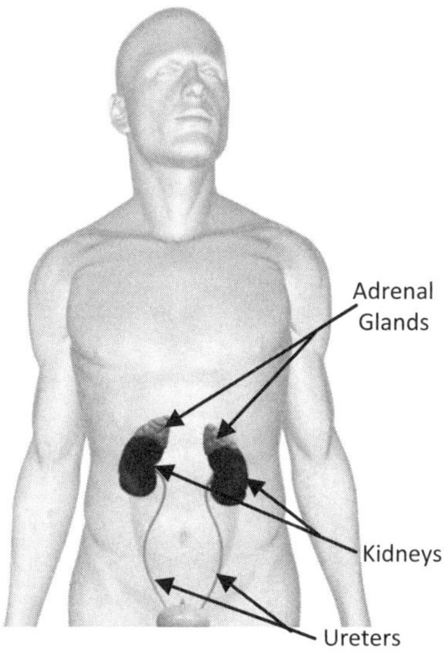

Prostate Problems

Prostate problems have many potential causes, however what follows are the basic mechanics. The Kidney/Adrenal system produces raw materials for the production of hormones (for example, testosterone) the body uses to control many functions, including reproductive organ and gland function.

Kidney/Adrenal system malfunction can cause many problems with the prostate, including swelling and/or enlargement, thus negatively affecting reproductive function and/or urination.

As you can see with this particular health problem, there is an underlying cause. The key to success in treating these problems lies in addressing the underlying issue described above to eliminate the problem over the long term. To speed Acupuncture and/or Chinese Herbal Medicine results, it is recommended one minimally reduce or eliminate the intake of caffeine, beer, deep-fried foods, dairy, sugar, preservatives in food, chemicals in food and municipal tap water (which most often contains chlorine and fluoride, considered by many as dangerous chemicals

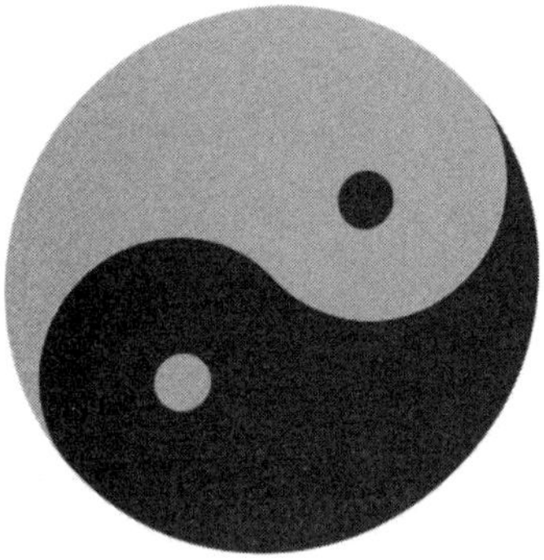

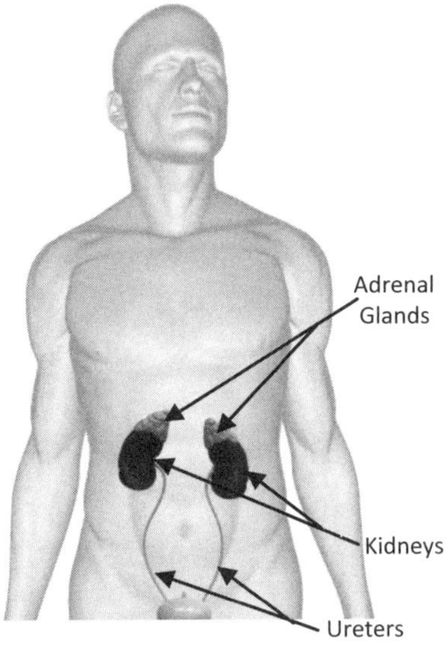

Restless Leg Syndrome

Restless leg syndrome has many potential causes, however what follows are the basic mechanics. The Kidney/Adrenal system is the root of the "yin" and the "yang" of the body. (See diagram above on the left.) The yin of the body is cool, moist, and nourishing (an example of yin in the body would be the amniotic fluid around a baby). The yang of the body is hot, moving, and invigorating (an example of yang in the body would be a woman experiencing hot flashes where the yang goes "awry"). A deficiency of yin will cause the yang to "rise" at the most yin time of the day (night), causing the muscles to become active when they are supposed to be relaxed and immobile.

As a person goes through life, there are a variety of stressors that can cause a loss of Kidney/Adrenal function. As that function begins to slip, the yin of the Kidney/Adrenal system may become depleted, causing the yang to become overactive, over-stimulating the muscles of the legs.

As you can see with this particular health problem, there is an underlying cause. The key to success in treating these problems lies in addressing the underlying issue described above to eliminate the problem over the long term. To speed Acupuncture and/or Chinese Herbal Medicine results, it is recommended one minimally reduce or eliminate the intake of caffeine, beer, deep-fried foods, dairy, sugar, preservatives in food, chemicals in food and municipal tap water (which most often contains chlorine and fluoride, considered by many as dangerous chemicals).

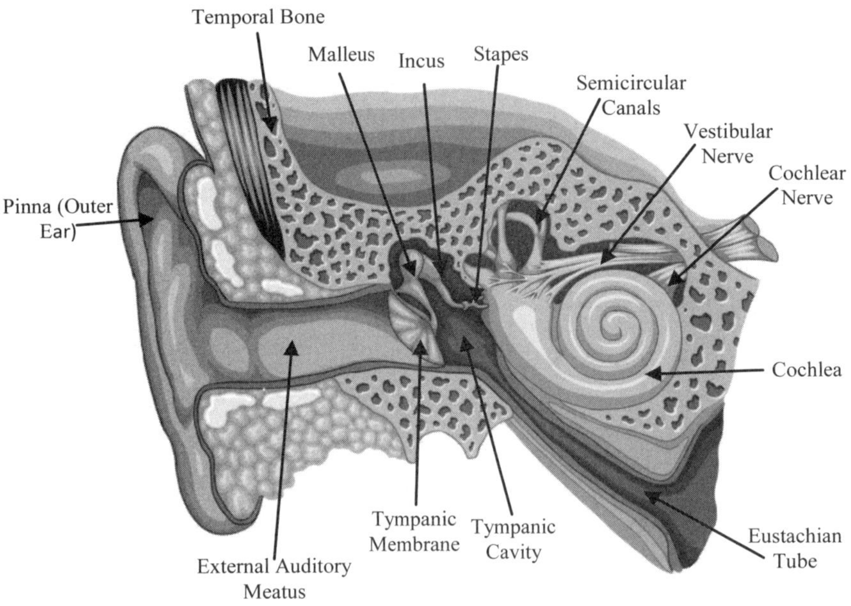

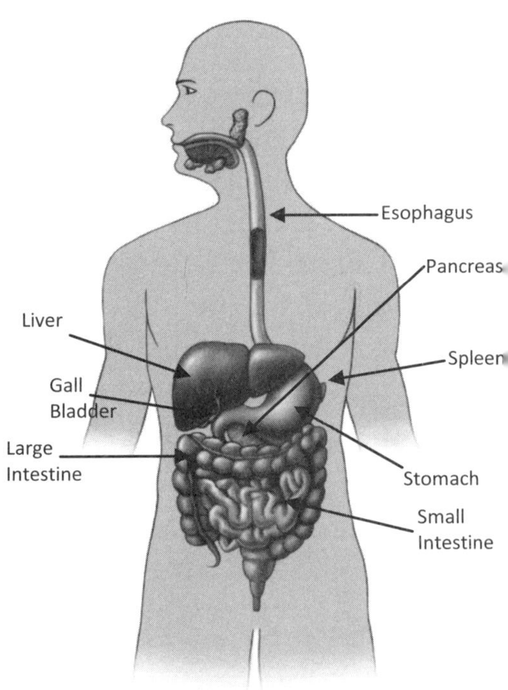

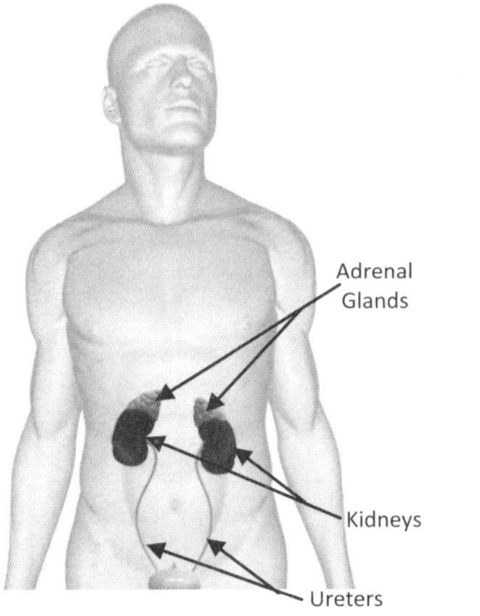

Ringing in the Ears

Ringing in the ears has three potential causes.

1. Kidney/Adrenal system is related to the function of the ears. A loss of Kidney/Adrenal system function may cause low-pitched ringing in the ears.

2. High-pitched ringing in the ears may be caused by a breakdown in Liver function. Of the Liver's 600 physiological functions, one of which

is to help the body adapt to the mental and emotional stresses of life. In other words, if one's Liver is functioning at a high level, stress entering one's life has no physical effect; however, if one's Liver isn't functioning well, stress can have a negative effect on the body, including constricting the blood vessels which may cause high-pitched ringing in the ears.

3. Inner ear structural damage from the sound waves of intensely loud noise may also cause ringing in the ears (for example, in cases of airplane mechanics or musicians who do not use ear plugs).

Given that one of the Liver's 600 functions is to purify the bloodstream, reducing or eliminating the intake of toxic chemicals is very important as part of a larger strategy to resolve ringing in the ears. It is also important to exercise vigorously (to a point of perspiration) for at least 30 minutes four times weekly, thus increasing Liver circulation, soothing the Liver and stimulating increased circulation throughout the body, which allows the body to detoxify at least to a small degree.

As you can see with this particular health problem, there is an underlying cause. The key to success in treating these problems lies in addressing the underlying issue described above to eliminate the problem over the long term. To speed Acupuncture and/or Chinese Herbal Medicine results, it is recommended one minimally reduce or eliminate the intake of caffeine, deep-fried foods, dairy, sugar, preservatives in food, chemicals in food and municipal tap water (which most often contains chlorine and fluoride, considered by many as dangerous chemicals).

Sciatica/Hip Pain

Sciatica and hip pain have many potential causes, however what follows are the four basic possibilities:

1. Trauma or injury can cause a problem with blood, nerve, and/or energy circulation in the lower back, leading to pain that radiates into the buttocks and/or leg. Scar tissue may result, complicating the condition (see section "Pain due to Scar Tissue").

2. Kidney/Adrenal system governs the function and structure of the lower back. If the Kidney/Adrenal system function declines, they may shrink (perhaps as little as several millimeters) causing the surrounding muscle tissue to fill the resulting space. Such muscle changes may, in turn, cut off circulation and/or pull the spine's vertebral bones out of place, causing an impingement of the nerve and pain. Nerve damage in any part of the body may often cause a person to experience strange, shooting pains.

3. Reduced energy circulation locally may cause dull pain.

4. Lack of blood circulation may cause sharp pain.

Any or all of the above may be involved when one experiences sciatica and/or hip pain.

As you can see with this particular health problem, there is an underlying cause. The key to success in treating these problems lies in addressing the underlying issue described above to eliminate the problem over the long term. To speed Acupuncture and/or Chinese Herbal Medicine results, it is recommended one minimally reduce or eliminate the intake of caffeine, deep-fried foods, dairy, sugar, preservatives in food, chemicals in food and municipal tap water (which most often contains chlorine and fluoride, considered by many as dangerous chemicals).

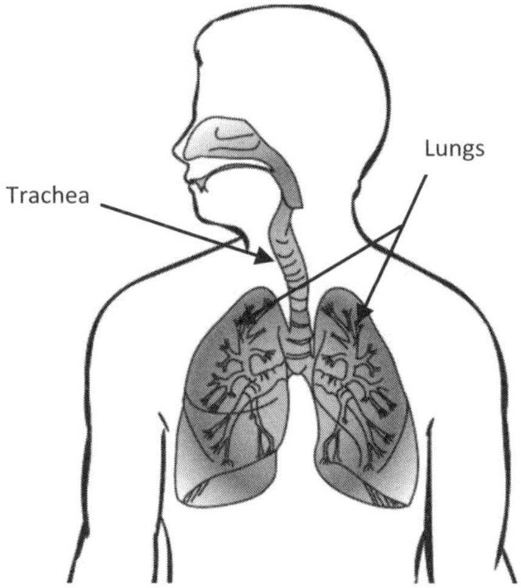

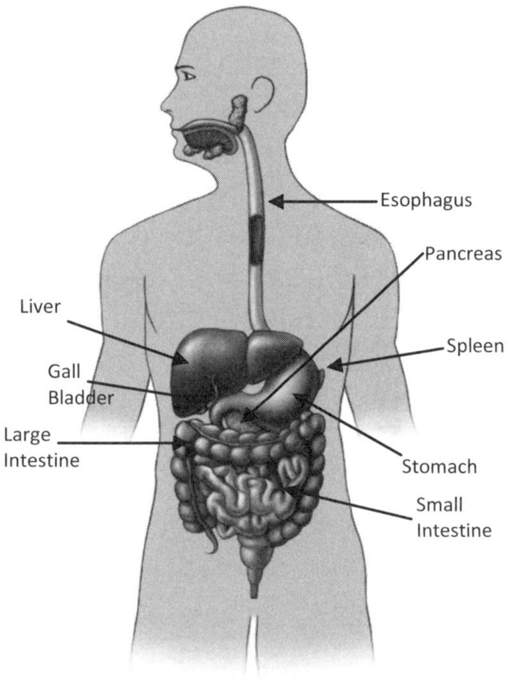

Shingles

Shingles may have many potential causes, however what follows are the basic mechanics.

The skin is governed by Liver and Lung function.

The herpes virus can attack the body in many ways, one of which is to attack the Liver and the nervous system, where it apparently may exist dormant for some time. Stress and other factors may then activate the virus, causing moisture-related skin problems (boils, oozing, etc) and attacking, causing potentially extreme discomfort.

Given that one of the Liver's 600 functions is to purify the bloodstream, reducing or eliminating the intake of toxic chemicals is very important as part of a larger strategy to resolve ringing in the ears. It is also important to exercise vigorously (to a point of perspiration) for at least 30 minutes four times weekly, thus increasing Liver circulation, soothing the Liver and stimulating increased circulation throughout the body, which allows the body to detoxify at least to a small degree.

As you can see with this particular health problem, there is an underlying cause. The key to success in treating these problems lies in addressing the underlying issue described above to eliminate the problem over the long term. To speed Acupuncture and/or Chinese Herbal Medicine results, it is recommended one minimally reduce or eliminate the intake of caffeine, deep-fried foods, dairy, sugar, preservatives in food, chemicals in food and municipal tap water (which most often contains chlorine and fluoride, considered by many as dangerous chemicals).

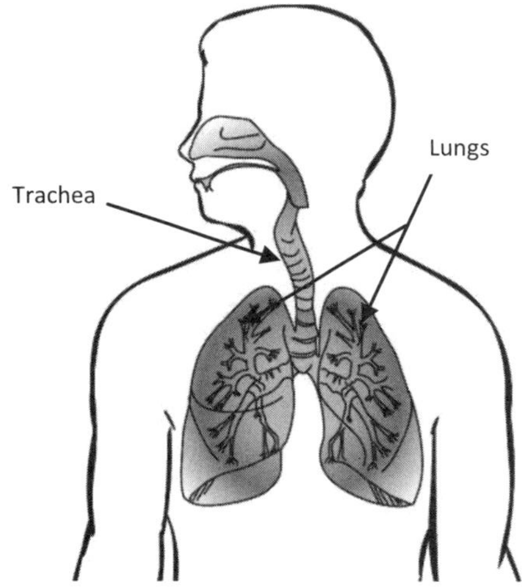

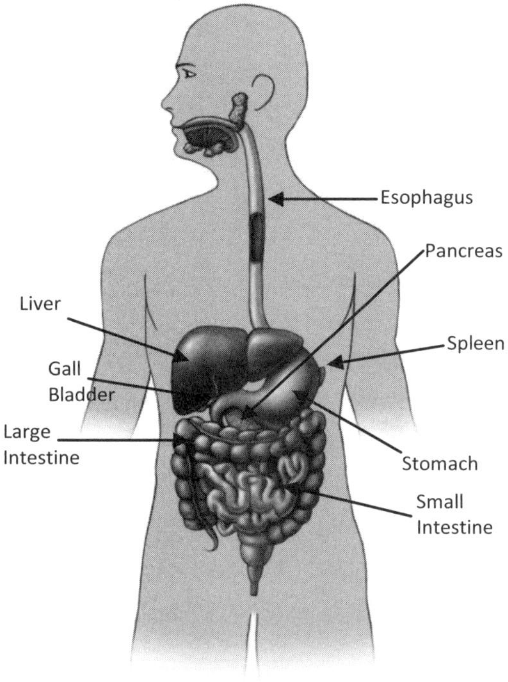

Sinus Problems

Sinus problems, such as nasal congestion or rhinitis (a runny nose) have many potential causes, however what follows are the basic mechanics. The Spleen and the Lungs govern the immune system and are involved in fluid metabolism and distribution, and although other systems in the body can be involved, these are most often involved with sinuses problems.

The Spleen, understood in Western Medicine as connected to the lymphatic system, transforms fluids in the body and generates internal immune system activity, fighting pathogens that penetrate deeper into the body and destroying pathogens in the blood stream to prevent sinus problems. If one were to eat or inhale a potential allergen, a well-functioning Spleen eliminates such material.

The Lungs, which open to the nose, throat, and sinuses, govern external immune function. If the sinuses and the Lungs are functioning well, the nasal mucosal membranes carry immune system factors that destroy incoming pathogenic material such as pollen.

The following 2,000-year-old quote helps to clarify further these organs role in immune function: *when the Spleen malfunctions it may cause fluids to accumulate in the body; when the Lungs malfunction they will take on those fluids.* An example of this would be one consuming food and fluids that that the Stomach and Spleen cannot fully metabolize. Those fluids will often "travel" upwards into the Lungs. The Lungs, to protect themselves, may activate the cilia (very fine hairs designed to move substances upwards out of the Lungs), which may likely push those fluids out of the Lungs and into the sinuses, causing sinus problems.

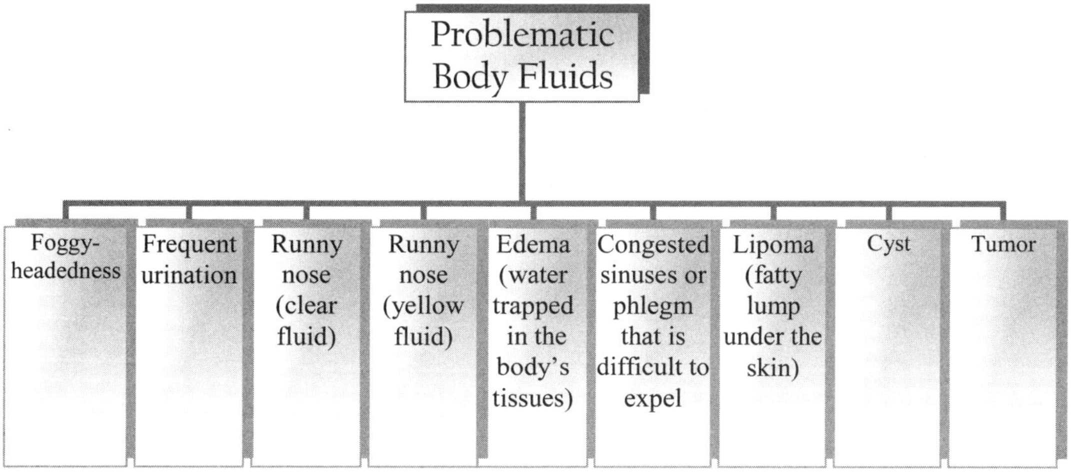

In Oriental Medicine there exists a scale (see above) that depicts fluids that are not fully metabolized or distributed appropriately, often caused by Kidney/Adrenal system, Spleen/Pancreatic system, or Lung malfunction.

At one end of this scale, one experiences the most subtle, invisible form of fluids: a feeling of "foggy-headedness" (a feeling as if one has cotton in one's head), perhaps experienced on a rainy day. Further to the right on the scale, one may experience frequent urination. A bit further over on the scale, one experiences a runny nose with clear fluid. Further to the right one experiences nasal discharge with thick, yellow fluids. A little further to the right, one experience symptoms such as edema: swollen ankles, abdominal bloating, and/or inflamed sinuses with fluids underneath the surface of the mucus membranes. Even further to the right, one may experience a small lipoma (a soft, round or oval deposit of fatty material that grows under the skin). Further to the right still, a cyst; and finally, at the extreme right end of the scale would be a tumor that is fixed in location, dense, and potentially dangerous.

As you can see with this particular health problem, there is an underlying cause. The key to success in treating these problems lies in addressing the underlying issue described above to eliminate the problem over the long term. To speed Acupuncture and/or Chinese Herbal Medicine results, it is recommended one minimally reduce or eliminate the intake of caffeine, deep-fried foods, dairy, sugar, preservatives in food, chemicals in food and municipal tap water (which most often contains chlorine and fluoride, considered by many as dangerous chemicals).

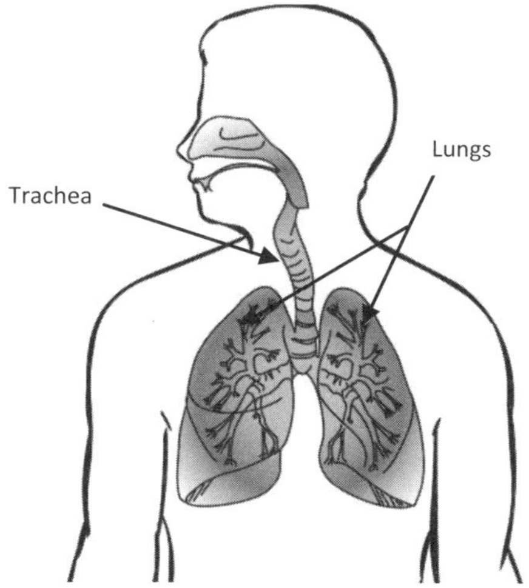

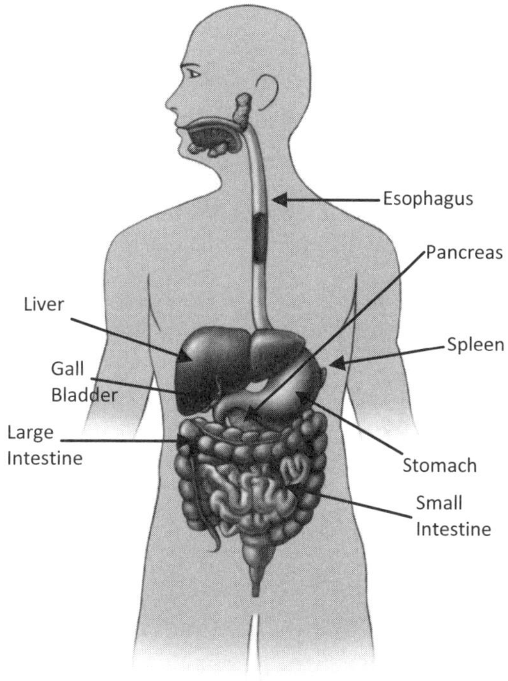

Skin Conditions

Skin conditions have many potential causes, however what follows are the basic mechanics. The skin has 32 layers, between which toxins may become caught (to imagine these layers and the material that may exist between them, picture many grains of sand stuck between 32 layers of paper).

The Liver and Lungs govern skin function; if the Liver and/or Lung malfunction, it can be difficult for them to nourish all of the layers of skin.

<u>Moisture-Related Skin Conditions</u>

Toxins and/or "heat" (from chemicals in food, alcohol, drugs, etc.) may accumulate in the body's fatty tissue and/or organ system. When released from the tissue, those toxins may cause moisture-related skin problems (involving boils, oozing, etc) with Liver or Lung system malfunction, rather than being eliminated via the bowel movements and/or urination, the most ideal elimination routes.

Conversely, rapid exposure to extraordinary amounts of toxins may cause the Liver and Lung to efficiently eliminate all of those toxins via the skin as an additional route (in addition to the bowel movement and urination).

Dry Skin Conditions

Red, dry, cracking, or peeling skin indicates the Lung and/or Liver systems are unable to nourish the skin.

Toxins and/or "heat" caused by many factors may also dry the skin, causing such symptoms.

Given that one of the Liver's 600 functions is to purify the bloodstream, reducing or eliminating the intake of toxic chemicals is very important as part of a larger strategy to resolve most skin conditions. It is also important to exercise vigorously (to a point of perspiration) for at least 30 minutes four times weekly, thus increasing Liver circulation, soothing the Liver and stimulating increased circulation throughout the body, which allows the body to detoxify at least to a small degree.

As you can see with this particular health problem, there is an underlying cause. The key to success in treating these problems lies in addressing the underlying issue described above to eliminate the problem over the long term. To speed Acupuncture and/or Chinese Herbal Medicine results, it is recommended to use organic, chemical-free moisturizers; organic, chemical-free soaps; organic, chemical-free shampoos, to filter shower and bath water to remove chlorine and to use supplements such as vitamin E, evening primrose oil and vitamin B-2, all of which build skin function. Additionally, it is recommended minimally to reduce or eliminate the intake of caffeine, deep-fried foods, dairy, sugar, preservatives in food, chemicals in food and municipal tap water (which most often contains chlorine and fluoride, considered by many as dangerous chemicals).

Smoking Cessation

There are five different addiction centers in the brain that are affected by cigarette smoking, making it more addictive than heroine. Smoking negatively affects all of the vital organs, but most significantly the Lungs, the Heart, and the Liver.

Smoking's most significant problem is high-volume chemical inhalation, however even chemical-free cigarettes cause a drying effect in the Lungs and other body tissues.

To break this particular type of addiction, one need implement a comprehensive program, including Acupuncture, dietary changes and possibly Chinese Herbal Medicine. Additionally, it is important to exercise vigorously (to a point of perspiration) for at least 30 minutes four times weekly, thus increasing Liver circulation, soothing the Liver and stimulating increased circulation throughout the body, which allows the body to detoxify at least to a small degree.

As you can see with this particular health problem, there is an underlying cause. The key to success in treating these problems lies in addressing the underlying issue described above to eliminate the problem over the long term. To speed Acupuncture and/or Chinese Herbal Medicine results, it is recommended one minimally reduce or eliminate the intake of caffeine, deep-fried foods, dairy, sugar, preservatives in food, chemicals in food and municipal tap water (which most often contains chlorine and fluoride, considered by many as dangerous chemicals). Upon discontinuing this addiction, it is vital to de-acidify the body.

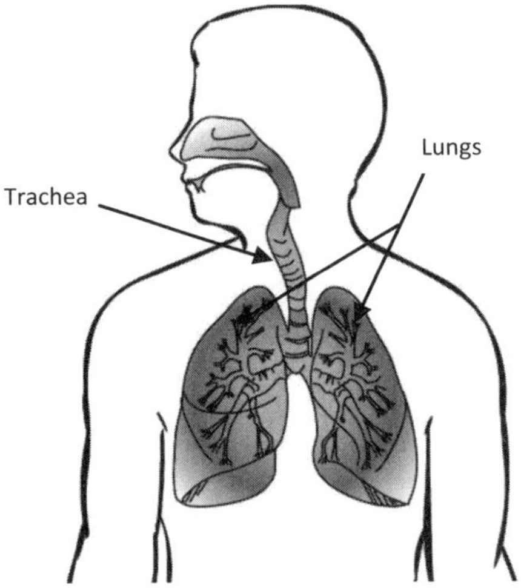

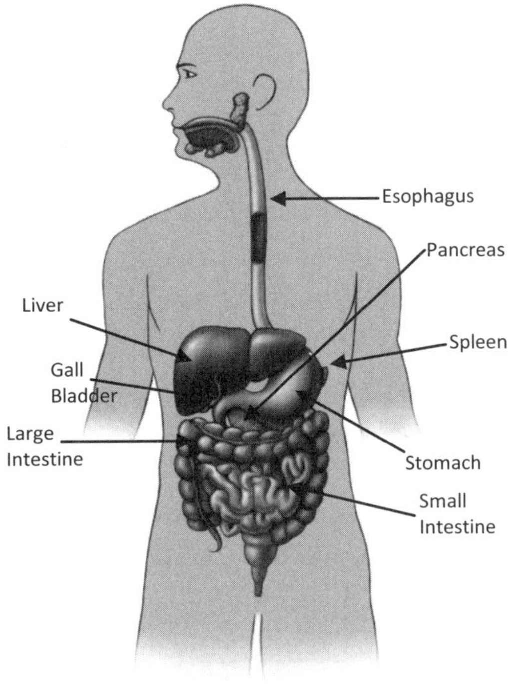

Snoring

Snoring has many potential causes, however what follows are the basic mechanics.

The Spleen and the Lungs are most often involved with fluid metabolism and distribution, therefore they are usually involved with sinus problems such as snoring to some degree although other systems in the body may be involved.

The Spleen, understood in Western Medicine as connected to the lymphatic system, transforms fluids in the body.

The Lungs--which open to the nose, throat, and sinuses--are often involved with sinus issues such as snoring.

The following 2,000-year-old quote helps to clarify further these organs role with sinus problems such as snoring: *when the Spleen malfunctions it may cause fluids to accumulate in the body; when the Lungs malfunction they will take on those fluids.* An example of this would be one consuming food and fluids that that the Stomach and Spleen cannot fully metabolize. Those fluids will often "travel" upwards into the Lungs. The Lungs, to protect themselves, may activate the cilia (very fine hairs designed to move substances upwards out of the Lungs), which may likely push those fluids out of the Lungs and into the sinuses, causing air to travel through the fluids, causing oftentimes loud sounds. As one lays horizontally, gravity does not move those fluids down again into the Lungs.

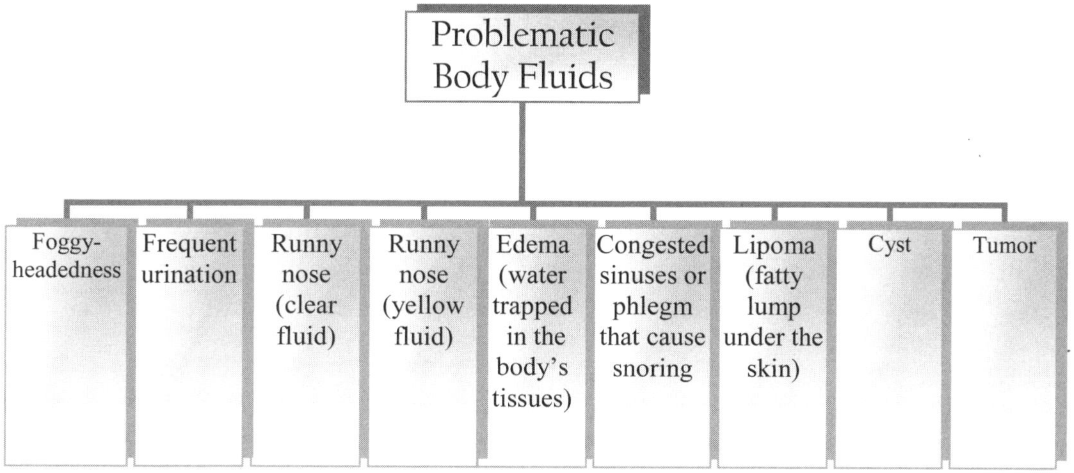

In Oriental Medicine there exists a scale (see above) that depicts fluids that are not fully metabolized or distributed appropriately, often caused by Kidney/Adrenal system, Spleen/Pancreatic system, or Lung malfunction.

At one end of this scale, one experiences the most subtle, invisible form of fluids: a feeling of "foggy-headedness" (a feeling as if one has cotton in one's head), perhaps experienced on a rainy day. Further to the right on the scale, one may experience frequent urination. A bit further over on the scale, one experiences a runny nose with clear fluid. Further to the right one experiences nasal discharge with thick, yellow fluids. If those fluids become congested, they may lead to snoring. A little further to the right, one experience symptoms such as edema: swollen ankles, abdominal bloating, and/or inflamed sinuses with fluids underneath the surface of the mucus membranes. Even further to the right, one may experience a small lipoma (a soft, round or oval deposit of fatty material that grows under the skin). Further to the right still, a cyst; and finally, at the extreme right end of the scale would be a tumor that is fixed in location, dense, and potentially dangerous.

As you can see with this particular health problem, there is an underlying cause. The key to success in treating these problems lies in addressing the underlying issue described above to eliminate the problem over the long term. To speed Acupuncture and/or Chinese Herbal Medicine results, it is recommended one minimally reduce or eliminate the intake of caffeine, deep-fried foods, dairy, sugar, preservatives in food, chemicals in food and municipal tap water (which most often contains chlorine and fluoride, considered by many as dangerous chemicals).

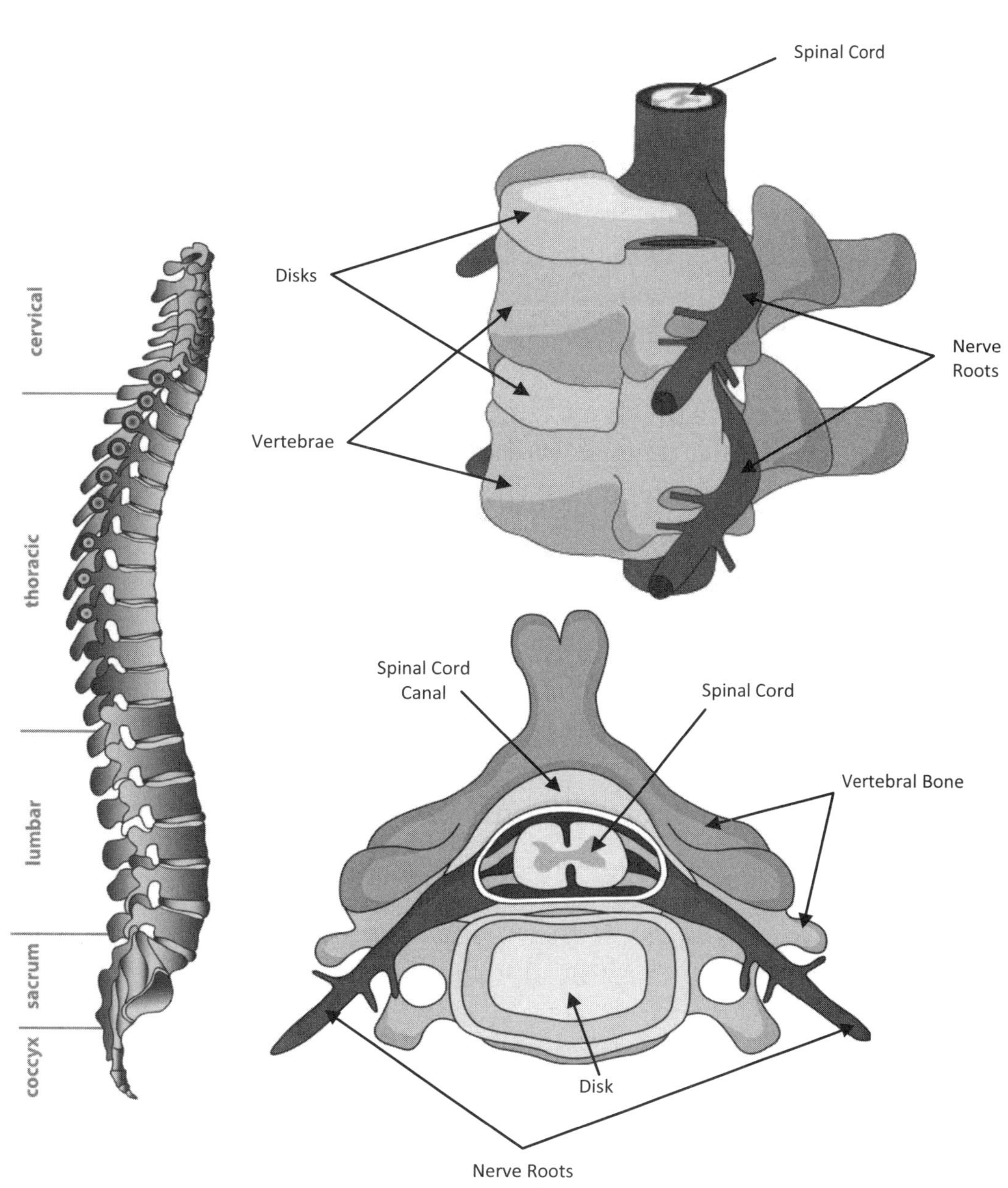

Spinal Column Disk Problems

Spinal column disk problems have many potential causes, however what follows are the basic mechanics.

The Kidney/Adrenal system governs the function of the bones and, therefore the vertebrae (bones of the spine). Kidney/Adrenal system also governs the function and structure of the lower back. If the Kidney/Adrenal system function declines, they may shrink (perhaps as little as several millimeters) causing the surrounding muscle tissue to fill the resulting space. Such muscle changes may, in turn, cut off circulation and/or pull the spine's vertebral bones out of place, causing an impingement of the nerve and pain.

The Liver system is involved with spinal disk function. The disks provide a cushion intended to move and flex depending on the body's activity. Nerves, connected to the spinal cord, originate in the space between the vertebrae and disks. If the disk shape becomes abnormal, the vertebrae can then pinch the nerves which cause problems, including pain that may refer to many places on the body. It can then affect blood flow and energy flow causing muscle spasms, referred pain, and so on.

The disks may be affected in several ways, including a mild nerve impingement, a disk "slip" or herniation (a condition in which the center of the disk bulges out of its normal shape), or a disk rupture (the disk bursting).

Acupuncture drives blood and energy into the disk so it may begin to function normally. Acupuncture also gets the muscles in the area functioning normally and, thus strengthened, they again naturally separate the two vertebrae, allowing the disk to resume its normal shape.

As you can see with this particular health problem, there is an underlying cause. The key to success in treating these problems lies in addressing the underlying issue described above to eliminate the problem over the long term. To speed Acupuncture and/or Chinese Herbal Medicine results, it is recommended one minimally reduce or eliminate the intake of caffeine, deep-fried foods, dairy, sugar, preservatives in food, chemicals in food and municipal tap water (which most often contains chlorine and fluoride, considered by many as dangerous chemicals).

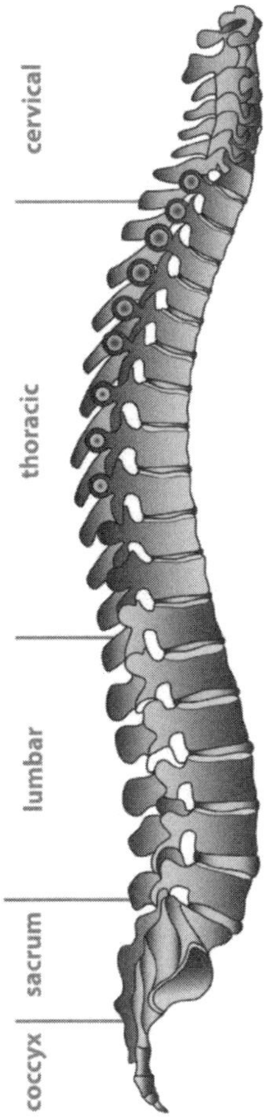

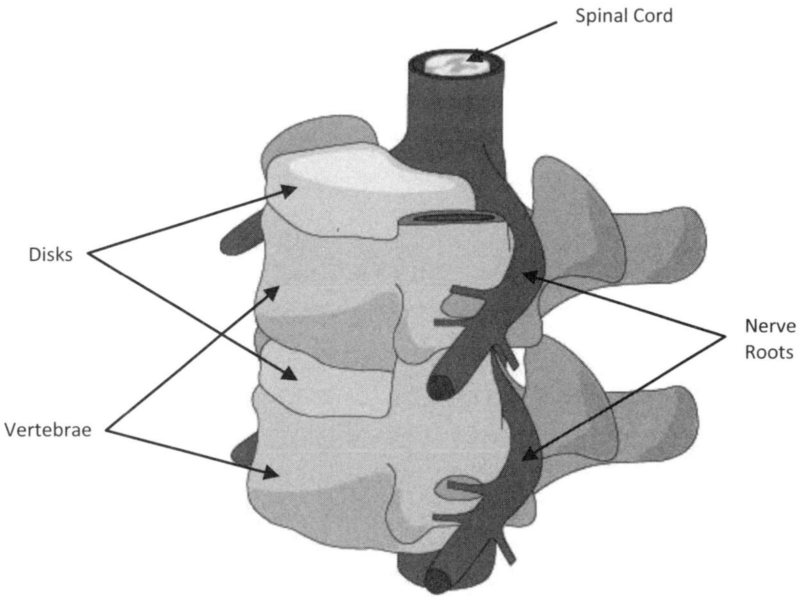

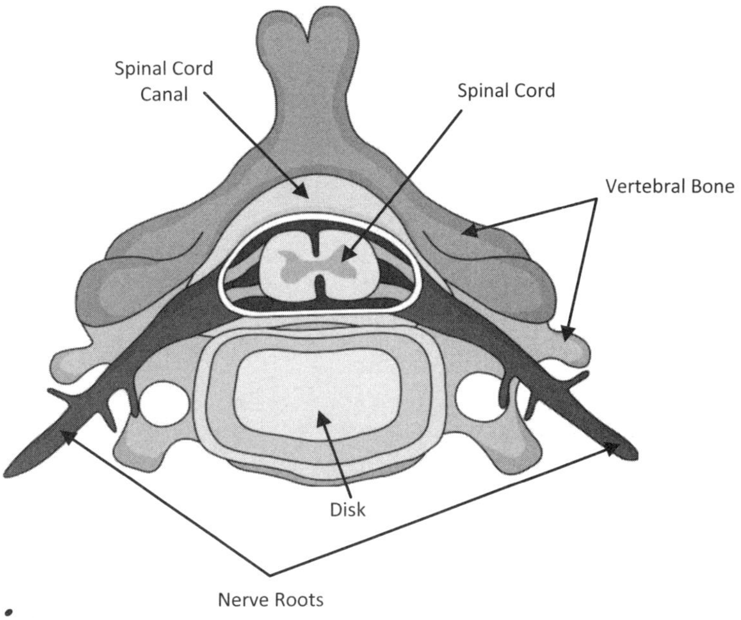

Spinal Stenosis

Spinal stenosis (narrowing of the spinal canal, which is the space in the center of the vertebrae, through which the spinal cord travels) has many potential causes, however what follows are the basic mechanics. The Kidney/Adrenal system governs the function of the bones and therefore the vertebrae (bones of the spine). The Liver system governs the function of the disks between the vertebrae.

The vertebrae may be affected in several ways, including stenosis.

Acupuncture drives blood and energy into the spine so it may begin to function normally, thereby changing the structure of the spinal canal, increasing the space the spinal cord requires for proper function and potentially decreasing inflammation. Obviously, it is ideal to avoid spinal surgery, if at all possible.

As you can see with this particular health problem, there is an underlying cause. The key to success in treating these problems lies in addressing the underlying issue described above to eliminate the problem over the long term. To speed Acupuncture and/or Chinese Herbal Medicine results, it is recommended one minimally reduce or eliminate the intake of caffeine, deep-fried foods, dairy, sugar, preservatives in food, chemicals in food and municipal tap water (which most often contains chlorine and fluoride, considered by many as dangerous chemicals).

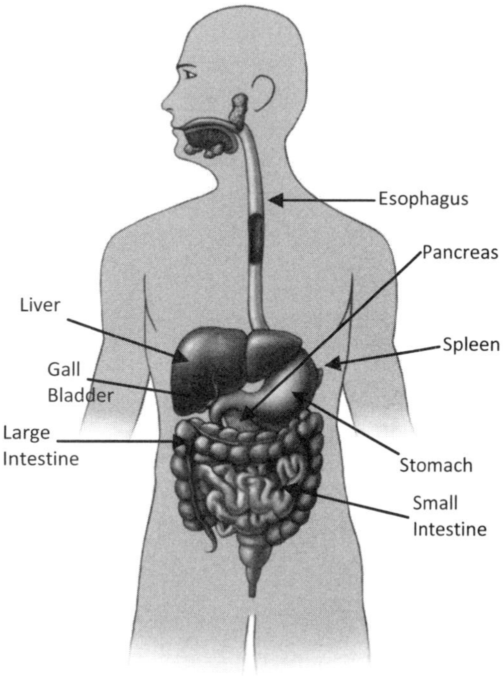

Stress, Difficulty Adapting to

Difficulty adapting to stress has many potential causes, however what follows are the basic mechanics. Thousands of years ago, physicians in China began to explore the nature of human emotion and discovered a direct link between emotion and the organ system. Having helped many people resolve emotional imbalances over the years, we've found the following to be accurate from the point of view of the physical body (obviously many factors exist in life that may trigger bodily malfunction which, in turn, could then trigger an emotional response). What is described below is the relationship between the emotions and physical body.

The Liver has 600 physiological functions, one of which is to help the body adapt to the mental and emotional stresses of life. In other words, if one's Liver is functioning at a high level, stress entering one's life has no physical effect; however, if one's Liver isn't functioning well, stress can have a negative effect on the body.

Liver malfunction can cause a person to experience difficulty adapting to stress, excessive or inappropriate anger, irritability, frustration, impatience, and/or depression. For example, a person with multiple emotional stresses over many years may experience suppressed Liver function. Then, the loss of a loved one could cause Liver function to drop dramatically, and the person could then begin to experience difficulty adapting to stress. On the other hand, a well-functioning Liver will cause one to be emotionally even and generally happy.

Difficulty adapting to stress can be caused by a breakdown in Liver function, not simply an imbalance in brain chemistry (the typical Western Medical view of this particular condition). Ironically, addressing only the brain chemistry with medication often leads to further difficulty resolving the problem as shown here: if one takes a medication for "stress" (which may be caused by a Liver imbalance) and that medication reduces Liver function (the Liver, in its capacity as a blood purifier, will attempt to eliminate the chemical from the body), it makes it more difficult to treat the problem. This explains why a person may take a medication their entire life.....and the issues never fully resolves!

Given that one of the Liver's 600 functions is to purify the bloodstream, reducing or eliminating the intake of toxic chemicals is very important as part of a larger strategy to resolve difficulty adapting to stress. It is also important to exercise vigorously (to a point of perspiration) for at least 30 minutes four times weekly, thus increasing Liver circulation, soothing the Liver and stimulating increased circulation throughout the body, which allows the body to detoxify at least to a small degree.

As you can see with this particular health problem, there is an underlying cause. The key to success in treating these problems lies in addressing the underlying issue described above to eliminate the problem over the long term. To speed Acupuncture and/or Chinese Herbal Medicine results, it is recommended one minimally reduce or eliminate the intake of caffeine, deep-fried foods, dairy, sugar, preservatives in food, chemicals in food and municipal tap water (which most often contains chlorine and fluoride, considered by many as dangerous chemicals).

Tendonitis

Tendonitis has many potential causes, however what follows are the basic mechanics. Tendonitis involves inflammation of the tendons (tough cords of tissue that connect muscles to other tissues, such as bones).

The Liver governs the tendons and ligaments; a Liver imbalance may lead to tendon-based problems. Repetitive motion and/or physical trauma may cause the inflammation.

Using Acupuncture, the first step is to encourage circulation to re-route around the inflammation to reduce the pain and discomfort. Then, Acupuncture is ideally used to drive circulation into the area which carries the inflammation away from the region, returning the tendon to its normal state, eliminating the source of the pain.

As you can see with this particular health problem, there is an underlying cause. The key to success in treating these problems lies in addressing the underlying issue described above to eliminate the problem over the long term. To speed Acupuncture and/or Chinese Herbal Medicine results, it is recommended one minimally reduce or eliminate the intake of caffeine, deep-fried foods, dairy, sugar, preservatives in food, chemicals in food and municipal tap water (which most often contains chlorine and fluoride, considered by many as dangerous chemicals).

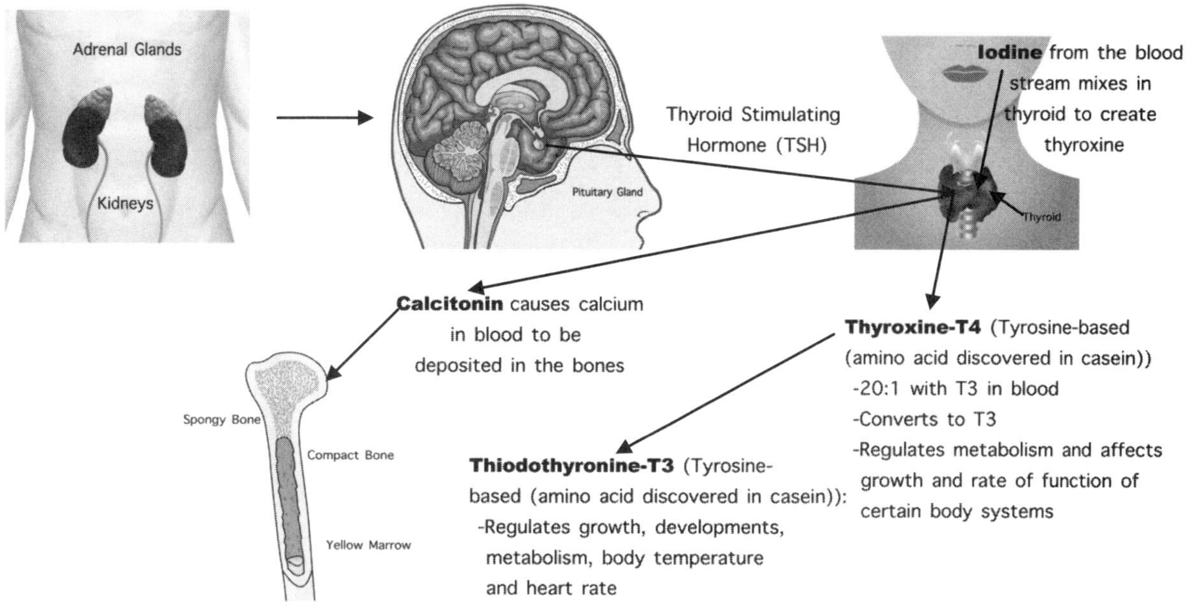

Thyroid Imbalances

Thyroid imbalances have many potential causes, however what follows are the basic mechanics. The Kidney/Adrenal system produces raw materials that stimulate glands (including the thyroid) to produce hormones that drive the endocrine system (the network of glands that produce secretions that drive many bodily functions). Too much or too little Kidney/Adrenal function can cause thyroid imbalances. The Thyroid is simply a superficial aspect of the problem.

Overall, the Thyroid controls the body's use of energy, the body's production of proteins and the body's sensitivity to other hormones in the following manner:

The Kidney/Adrenal system stimulates Pituitary gland function; in turn, the Pituitary gland releases Thyroid Stimulating Hormone (TSH) to the Thyroid, generating much of its function. Iodine from the blood stream is used by the Thyroid to create Thyroxin (known as T4, which regulates metabolism, growth and rate of function of other body systems);

eventually T4 converts in the bloodstream into Triiodothyronine (known as T3, which regulates growth, development, metabolism, body temperature and heart rate). The Thyroid also releases Calcitonin, which helps deposit calcium in the bloodstream into bone tissue.

In both Hypothyroid and Hyperthyroid conditions, one must regulate Thyroid function by normalizing the appropriate out-of-balance variable from the description above. Certain thyroid medications may cause the thyroid to atrophy: taking these medications for a period of time may cause the thyroid to shrink and lose function due to its inactivity. The longer period of time that one takes these medications, the less chance for the thyroid to recover, it seems.

As you can see with this particular health problem, there is an underlying cause. The key to success in treating these problems lies in addressing the underlying issue described above to eliminate the problem over the long term. To speed Acupuncture and/or Chinese Herbal Medicine results, it is recommended one minimally reduce or eliminate the intake of caffeine, deep-fried foods, dairy, sugar, preservatives in food, chemicals in food and municipal tap water (which most often contains chlorine and fluoride, considered by many as dangerous chemicals).

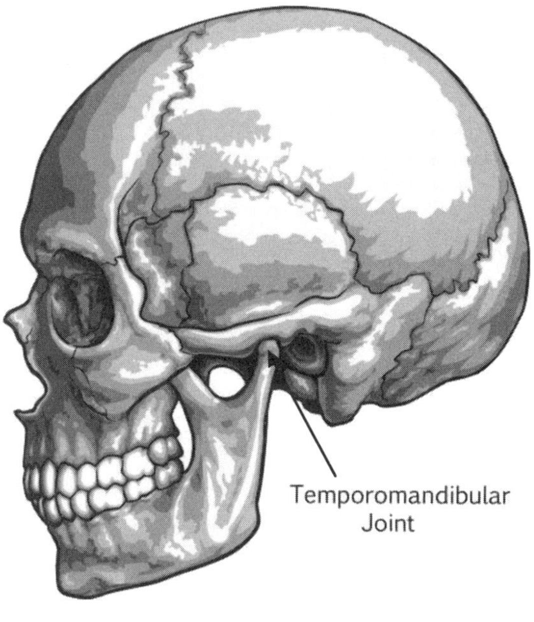

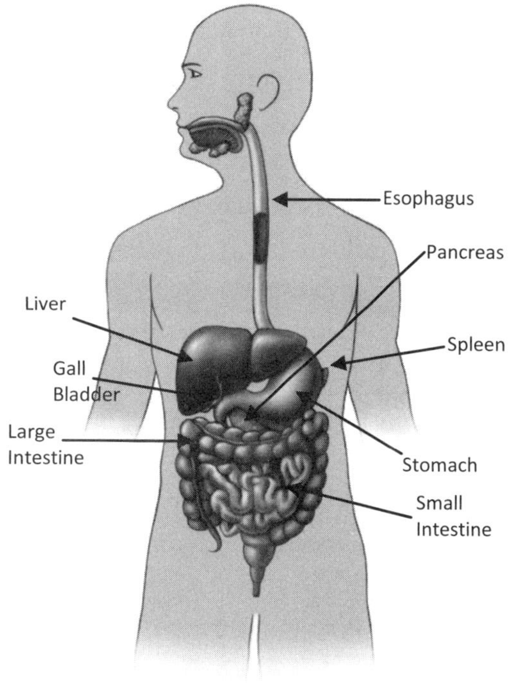

TMJ Syndrome

TMJ has many potential causes, however what follows are the basic mechanics. "Temporomandibular Joint Syndrome" refers to a variety of symptoms related to the area surrounding the jaw joint.

Thousands of years ago, physicians in China began to explore the nature of human emotion and discovered a direct link between emotion and the organ system.

The Liver has 600 physiological functions, one of which is to help the body adapt to life's mental and emotional stresses. In other words, if one's Liver is functioning at a high level, stress entering one's life has no physical effect, whereas if one's Liver isn't functioning well, stress can have a negative effect on the body. Another of the Liver's functions is to drive the blood and energy throughout the body, thereby causing the muscles to be relaxed.

Liver malfunction can cause a person to experience excessive or inappropriate anger, irritability, frustration, impatience, depression, and/or difficulty adapting to the mental/emotional stresses of life. For example, a person with multiple emotional stresses over many years may experience suppressed Liver function. The Liver may then reduce overall blood and energy circulation to the muscles (for example, in the jaw region), causing muscle constriction, pain and/or discomfort. On the other hand, a well-functioning Liver will cause one to be emotionally even and all of the body's muscles to be relaxed.

Difficulty adapting to life's stresses and muscle tension can be caused by a breakdown in Liver function, not simply a "structural" problem with the jaw. Often a person may use a splint (which can certainly be helpful to alleviate the symptoms of TMJ syndrome), however, the underlying cause of the TMJ may never fully resolve.

Given that one of the Liver's 600 functions is to purify the bloodstream, reducing or eliminating the intake of toxic chemicals is very important as part of a larger strategy to resolve difficulty adapting to stress and TMJ. It is also important to exercise vigorously (to a point of perspiration) for at least 30 minutes four times weekly, thus increasing Liver circulation, soothing the Liver and stimulating increased circulation throughout the body, which allows the body to detoxify at least to a small degree.

As you can see with this particular health problem, there is an underlying cause. The key to success in treating these problems lies in addressing the underlying issue described above to eliminate the problem over the long term. To speed Acupuncture and/or Chinese Herbal Medicine results, it is recommended one minimally reduce or eliminate the intake of caffeine, deep-fried foods, dairy, sugar, preservatives in food, chemicals in food and municipal tap water (which most often contains chlorine and fluoride, considered by many as dangerous chemicals

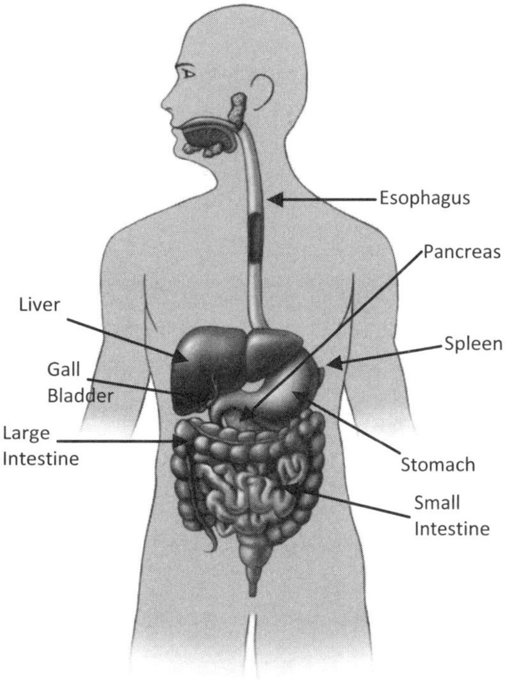

Tremors

Tremors ("Essential," "Familial," etc.) have many potential causes, however what follows are three possible causes, one or all of which may be involved:

1. Every muscle in the body requires a certain amount of blood circulation, delivering hormones, oxygen and nutrients such as potassium, calcium, etc. to the affected area. Muscles in the affected area may not receive adequate blood circulation, leading to involuntary movement.

2. Nervous system malfunction may cause abnormal muscle movement.

3. Liver malfunction may lead to abnormal muscle movement.

Given that one of the Liver's 600 functions is to purify the bloodstream, reducing or eliminating the intake of toxic chemicals is very important as part of a larger strategy to alleviating tremors. It is also important to exercise vigorously (if possible and with your doctor's supervision) to a point of perspiration for at least 30 minutes four times weekly, thus increasing Liver circulation, soothing the Liver and stimulating increased circulation throughout the body, which allows the body to detoxify at least to a small degree.

As you can see with this particular health problem, there is an underlying cause. The key to success in treating these problems lies in addressing the underlying issue described above to eliminate the problem over the long term. To speed Acupuncture and/or Chinese Herbal Medicine results, it is recommended one minimally reduce or eliminate the intake of caffeine, deep-fried foods, dairy, sugar, preservatives in food, chemicals in food and municipal tap water (which most often contains chlorine and fluoride, considered by many as dangerous chemicals).

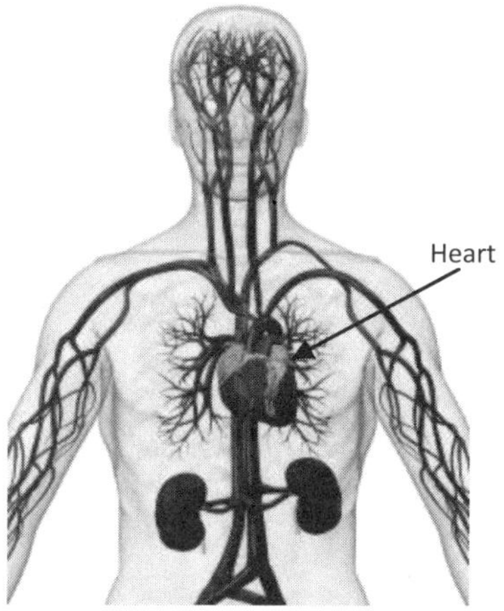

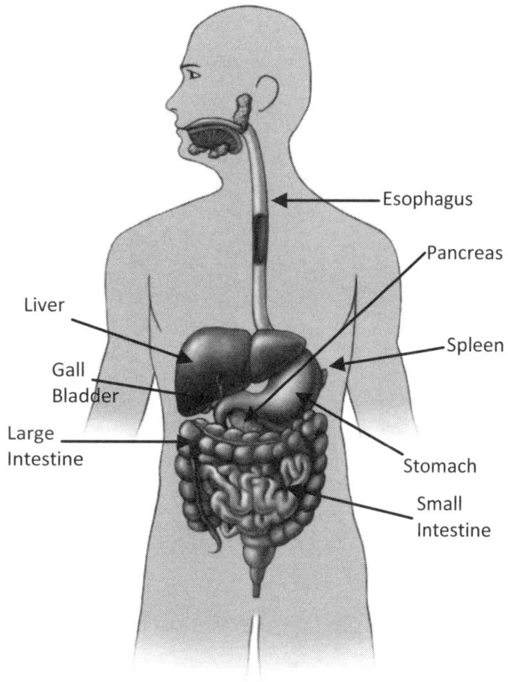

Varicose Veins

Varicose veins have many potential causes, however what follows are the basic mechanics at work. The Spleen/Pancreatic system governs the function and structure of the blood vessels and is also in charge of "suspending" the body's tissues (such as blood vessels) in place. Spleen/Pancreatic system malfunction may cause the veins to "float" to the surface of the skin and become visible, distended and/or painful.

As you can see with this particular health problem, there is an underlying cause. The key to success in treating these problems lies in addressing the underlying issue described above to eliminate the problem over the long term. To speed Acupuncture and/or Chinese Herbal Medicine results, it is recommended one minimally reduce or eliminate the intake of caffeine, deep-fried foods, dairy, sugar, preservatives in food, chemicals in food and municipal tap water (which most often contains chlorine and fluoride, considered by many as dangerous chemicals).

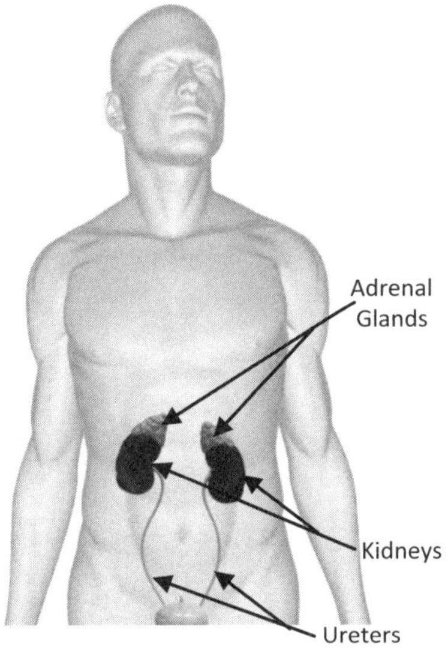

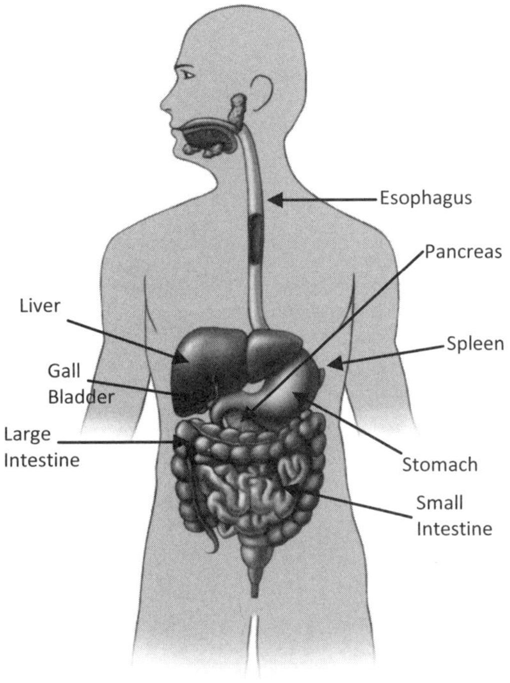

Weight Problems

Weight problems have many potential causes, however what follows are the basic mechanics. The Kidney/Adrenal system, the Spleen/Pancreatic system, and the Stomach govern the metabolism and may all be involved with weight problems.

The Kidney/Adrenal system is the root of the endocrine system, producing raw materials of hormones such as those that stimulate the Thyroid which, in turn, governs body temperature and metabolism.

The Spleen/Pancreatic system and the Stomach are largely responsible for breaking food and fluids down into useable nutrients, which are moved into the intestines and through the intestine wall into the blood stream to build, among other things, muscle tissue.

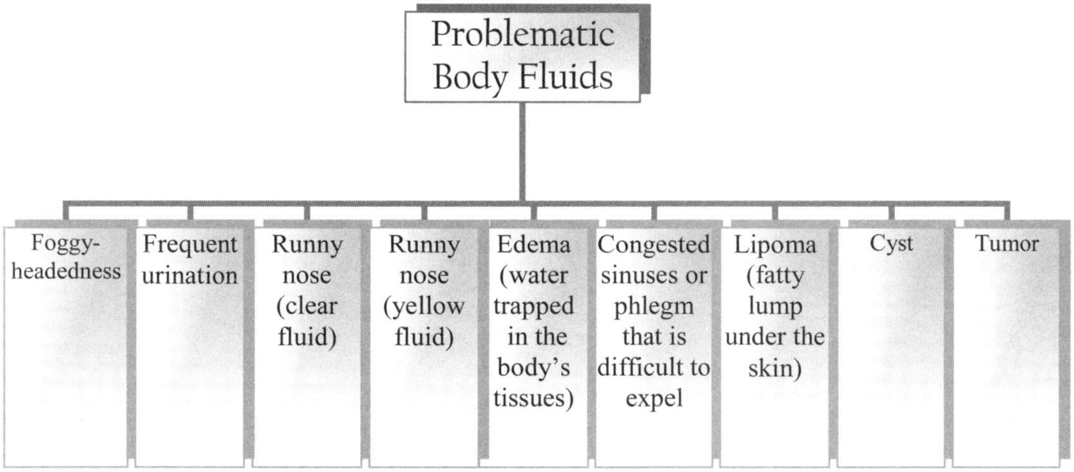

As you can see above, water weight (edema) and excess fatty tissue are both the result of inefficient metabolism.

It takes a broad spectrum of therapies to effectively treat weight problems, including exercise, nutrition, Acupuncture, and Chinese Herbal Medicine, all of which are necessary to effectively lose weight.

As you can see with this particular health problem, there is an underlying cause. The key to success in treating these problems lies in addressing the underlying issue described above to eliminate the problem over the long term. To speed Acupuncture and/or Chinese Herbal Medicine results, it is recommended one minimally reduce or eliminate the intake of items that can cause metabolic problems such as caffeine, deep-fried foods, raw foods, dairy, sugar, preservatives in food, chemicals in food and municipal tap water (which most often contains chlorine and fluoride, considered by many as dangerous chemicals).

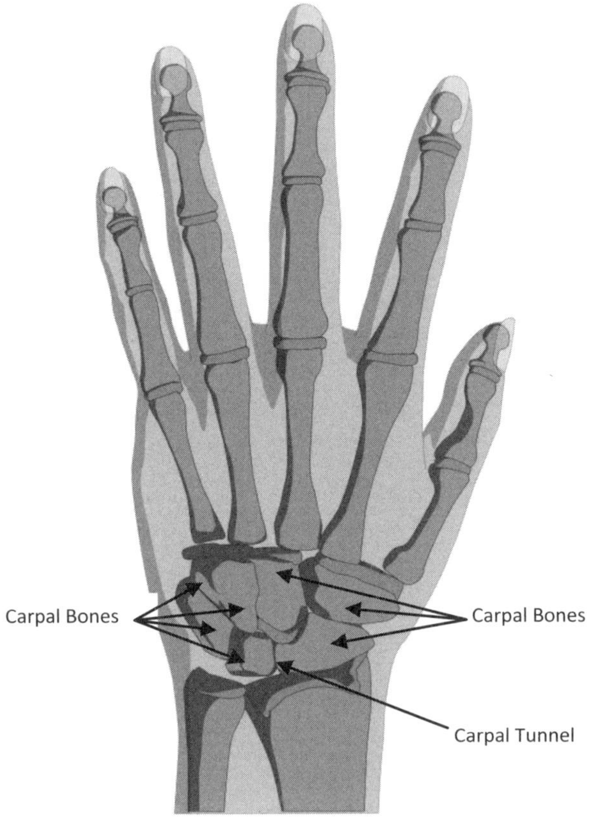

Wrist Pain

Wrist pain has many potential causes, however what follows are the basic mechanics.

Wrist pain may be caused by decreased blood and/or energy circulation in the affected area.

Specifically, carpal tunnel syndrome (the carpal tunnel is a passageway filled with ligaments, tendons, nerves, and bones at the base of the hand) may also be caused by:[8]

1. A lack of the body's nourishing fluids, wherein they are not lubricating the wrist joint properly (likened to an in adequately lubricated door hinge), causing pain.

---

[8] U.S. National Library of Medicine and National Institutes of Health, Carpal Tunnel Syndrome, http://www.nlm.nih.gov/medlineplus/carpaltunnelsyndrome.html (Accessed December, 2010)

2. A thickening from irritated tendons.

3. Swelling of other tissues that cause the nerve to be compressed.

As you can see with this particular health problem, there is an underlying cause. The key to success in treating these problems lies in addressing the underlying issue described above to eliminate the problem over the long term. To speed Acupuncture and/or Chinese Herbal Medicine results, it is recommended one minimally reduce or eliminate the intake of caffeine, deep-fried foods, dairy, sugar, preservatives in food, chemicals in food and municipal tap water (which most often contains chlorine and fluoride, considered by many as dangerous chemicals).

Image Credits:

Acupuncture Meridians of the Body, Front and Back
©Jun He, 2010 Used under license from Dreamstime.com

Acupuncture Meridians of the head
© Cammeraydave, 2010 Used under license from Dreamstime.com

Acupuncture Meridians of the Lower Back
©Jun He, 2010 Used under license from Dreamstime.com

Acupuncture Meridians of the Upper Back, Shoulder and Neck
©Spark067, Used under license from Dreamstime.com

Cardiovascular System
©Eraxion, 2010 Used under license from iStockphoto.com

Female Reproductive System
©Dee-jay, 2010 Used under license from iStockphoto.com

Five Elements
© Laura Patino, 2010

Full Spine
©Maryna Melnyk, 2010 Used under license from Shutterstock.com

Human Bone
©Cudazi, 2010 Used under license from Dreamstime.com

Human Brain
©Oguzaral, 2010 Used under license from Dreamstime.com

Human Digestive System
©Andrea Danti, 2010 Used under license from Shutterstock.com

Human Ear
©Oguz Aral, 2010 Used under license from Shutterstock.com

Human Eye
©Cafillu, 2010 Used under license from iStockphoto.com

Internal Organs
©Skalapendra, 2010 Used under license from Shutterstock.com

Male Urinary System
©Sebastian Kaulitzki, 2010 Used under license from Shutterstock.com

Prostate Gland Section Diagram
©IgorZakowski, 2010 Used under license from iStockphoto.com

Respiratory System
©Hkannn, 2010 Used under license from Shutterstock.com

Skull
©Oguzaral, 2010 Used under license from iStockphoto.com

Thyroid Gland
©Guniita, 2010 Used under license from Dreamstime.com

Vertebra Spinal Disc
©Mmutlu, 2010 Used under license from Shutterstock.com

Vertebra Disc-Top View
©Mmutlu, 2010 Used under license from Shutterstock.com

Wrist
©Sebastian Kaulitzki, 2010 Used under license from Shutterstock.com

YinYang:
© Laura Patino, 2010

Recommended Reading:

Beinfield, Harriet, and Korngold, Efrem, *Between Heaven and Earth: A Guide to Chinese Medicine*, New York: Ballentine Books, 1991. 431p.

Elias, Jason and Ketcham, Katherine, *The Five Elements of Self-Healing: Using Chinese Medicine for Maximum Immunity, Wellness, and Health*, Crown Publishing Group, 1998. 422p.

Kaptchuk, Ted, *The Web That Has No Weaver*, Chicago: NTC/Contemporary Publishing Group, 2000. 500p.

Maciocia, Giovanni, *The Foundations of Chinese Medicine*, New York: Churchhill Livingstone, 1989. 498p.

Tousley, John Dirk, *The Acupuncture Answer Book*, Laguna Beach: White Dove Publishing, 2009. 31p.

Find A Practitioner Near You:

I am happy to help! Simply contact me at either of the following addresses to find a local Acupuncturist who treats to improve function, not simply alleviate symptoms:

curry@milwaukeeacu.com
http://www.facebook.com/cchaudoir

Also, you can find a list of nationally certified Acupuncturists at:
www.nccaom.org

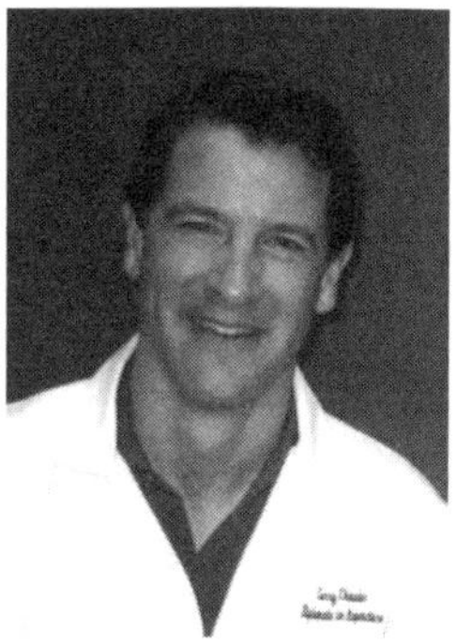

About the Author

Curry Chaudoir is the author of *Oriental Medicine and You: Making a Seemingly Complex, 3,500-year-old Medicine Understandable for the Layperson.* Chaudoir is an Acupuncturist and Executive Director of Acupuncture and Holistic Health Associates in Milwaukee, Wisconsin. He also teaches to Acupuncturists around the United States on a weekly basis.

He holds a BA from the University of Wisconsin-Milwaukee and a Master's of Science in Oriental Medicine from Southwest Acupuncture College in Santa Fe, New Mexico.

www.milwaukeeacu.com
curry@milwaukeeacu.com
http://www.facebook.com/cchaudoir

In his spare time he enjoys volleyball, camping, hiking and travel. He lives in Glendale, Wisconsin with his wife, April.

Index

abdominal gas/bloating, 26–27
acid reflux/heartburn, 28–29
acne, 30–31
Acupuncture
  for bursitis, 53
  for eye problems, 75–76
  method/purpose, 13
  for pain from scar tissue, 153–154
  for smoking cessation, 187
  for spinal column disk problems, 192
  for spinal column stenosis, 194
  for tendonitis, 198
  for weight problems, 207
ADD (Attention Deficit Disorder)/ADHD (Attention Deficit Hyperactivity Disorder), 45–46
addiction to smoking, 187
adrenal glands. *See* Kidney/Adrenal system
allergies, 32–35
anemia, 36
anger, 37–38
ankle/foot problems, 83, 148–149
anxiety, 39–40
arm pain, 148–149, 157–160. *See also* carpal tunnel syndrome
arthritis, 41–42
asthma, 43–44
Attention Deficit Disorder (ADD)/Attention Deficit Hyperactivity Disorder (ADHD), 45–46

back pain, 155–156, 159–160. *See also* spinal column
baldness, 87–88
Bell's Palsy, 47–49
"Bi" syndromes, 41
bladder. *See* Gall Bladder; Urinary Bladder
bloating/abdominal gas, 26–27
blood pressure
  high, 50–51, 92–94
  low, 51, 118–119
  systolic/diastolic numbers, 51–52, 92–93, 118–119
body fluids
  and cancer, 54–55, 82
  metabolism/distribution, 81–82, 207
  and sinus problems, 182–184
  and snoring, 188–190
body fluids (*cont.*)
  and weight problems, 206–207
brain chemistry, 63, 85, 114
bursitis, 53

cancer, 54–55, 82
carpal tunnel syndrome, 56–57, 208–209
Chinese Herbal Medicine, 13
cholesterol, 58–59
cigarette smoking, 187
circulation, 19–22, 51–52
  and exercise, 52, 90, 93–94
  and muscle cramping, 144
  and neuropathy, 148–149
  and pain, 155–156, 159–160
clotting, menstrual, 136–137
constipation, 60–61, 91
cramps
  menstrual/pre-menstrual, 138–139, 163–164
  muscle, 144

depression, 62–63
diabetes, 64–65, 148–149
diarrhea, 68–69
digestion, generally, 66–67, 165–167
diverticulitis, 70
dizziness/vertigo, 71–72
dysentery, 69

ears ringing, 176–177
earth element, 21, *21*, 24
edema, 81
elbow pain, 157–158
emotions. *See also* stress
  anger, 37–38
  anxiety, 39–40
  depression, 62–63
  frustration, 84–86
  irritability, 113–115
  mood swings, 130–131, 142–143, 168–170
Endometriosis, 73–74
exercise
  and cholesterol, 58–59
  and circulation, 52, 90, 93–94
  and Endometriosis, 73–74
  and Parkinson's disease, 161–162
eye problems, 75–76, 90, 141

fatigue, 77–78
fibromyalgia, 79–80
finger pain, 148–149
fire element, 21, *21*, 24
Five Element theory, 21, *21*, 24
fluids. *See* body fluids
foot/ankle problems, 83, 148–149
frustration, 84–86

Gall Bladder, 14
  functions, 17, 66
  headaches due to, 89–90, 140–141
glucose (sugar), 64–65

hair loss, 87–88
hand pain, 148–149
headaches, 75–76, 89–90, 140–141
Heart, 14
  and ADD/ADHD, 45–46
  and anxiety, 39
  and constipation, 61
  and fatigue, 78
  functions, 16
  and high blood pressure, 50–52, 93
  insomnia due to, 107, 109, 124, 126
  memory loss due to, 121
heartburn/acid reflux, 28–29
hemorrhoids, 91
Herbal Medicine, 13
herpes virus, 180–181
hip pain/sciatica, 178–179
hot flashes, 95, 122–123
hypothyroid (under-active thyroid)/hyperthyroid (over-active thyroid), 96–97, 199–200

immune function, 32–33, 43, 182–184
impotence, 98–99
incontinence, 100–102
infertility, 103–106
insomnia
  difficulty falling asleep, 107–108, 124–125
  waking during the night, 109–110, 126–127
  waking too early, 111–112, 128–129
insulin, 64–65
irritability, 113–115
Irritable Bowel Syndrome, 116–117

joint pain, 159–160

Kidney/Adrenal system, 14–15. *See also* yin and yang
  and abdominal gas/bloating, 26–27
  and ADD/ADHD, 45–46
  back pain due to, 155
  and bowel incontinence, 100
  and fatigue, 78
  and fibromyalgia, 79
  and fluid metabolism/distribution, 81
  functions, 16
  and hair loss, 87
  hip pain due to, 178
  and hot flashes, 95, 122–123
  and impotence, 98–99
  and infertility, 103, 105–106
  insomnia due to, 107–108, 110, 124–125, 127
  memory loss due to, 120
  narcolepsy due to, 146–147
  night sweats due to, 132–133, 150–151
  osteoporosis due to, 152
  prostate problems due to, 173
  restless leg syndrome due to, 174
  ringing in the ears due to, 176
  spinal column problems due to, 191–194
  and thyroid imbalances, 96–97, 199–200
  and urinary incontinence, 102
  vaginal dryness due to, 134–135
  and weight problems, 206

Large Intestine, 14
  and constipation, 60
  diarrhea due to, 68
  functions, 17, 66
legs
  pain in, 148–149, 159–160
  restless leg syndrome, 174–175
Liver, 14
  and acne, 30–31
  and anger, 37–38
  and Bell's Palsy, 47–48
  and cholesterol, 58–59
  and constipation, 60
  and depression, 62–63
  and digestion, 66–67, 165–166
  and dizziness/vertigo, 71–72
  and Endometriosis, 73–74
  eye problems due to, 75–76, 141
  and frustration, 84–85

Liver (*cont.*)
functions, 16, 66
headaches due to, 89–90, 140–141
and high blood pressure, 50–52, 93
insomnia due to, 109–111, 126, 128
irritability due to, 113–114
Irritable Bowel Syndrome due to, 116–117
menstrual clotting due to, 136–137
menstrual cramping due to, 138–139, 163–164
mood swings due to, 130–131, 142–143, 168–169
neck/shoulder pain due to, 157
and Parkinson's disease, 161–162
ringing in the ears due to, 176–177
and shingles, 180
skin conditions due to, 185–186
spinal column problems due to, 192
and stress, adapting to, 195–196
and strokes, 171–172
tendonitis due to, 198
TMJ due to, 201–202
and tremors, 203–204
Lungs, 14
and acne, 30
and allergies to airborne particles, 33
and asthma, 43
and fatigue, 77
and fluid metabolism/distribution, 81
functions, 16
narcolepsy due to, 146
and sinus problems, 182–184
skin conditions due to, 185–186
snoring due to, 188–190
lymphatic system, 182. *See also* Spleen/Pancreatic system

massage, 13
memory loss, 120–121
menopausal problems
hot flashes, 122–123
insomnia, 124–129
mood swings, 130–131, 168–170
night sweats, 132–133, 150–151
vaginal dryness, 134–135
menstrual problems
clotting, 136–137
cramping, 138–139, 163–164
digestive problems, 165–167
meridian system, 18
metal element, 21, *21*, 24
migraines, 75–76, 140–141
mood swings, 130–131, 142–143, 168–170
muscles
cramps, 144
and Parkinson's disease, 161–162
torn, 153–154
tremors, 203–204

narcolepsy, 145–147
nausea, 90, 141
neck pain, 157–158
neuropathy (disease of the nervous system), 148–149
numbness, 47–49, 83, 148, 159, 171
Nutrition, Oriental, 13

organ system, 13–18. *See also specific organs*
Oriental Medicine
branches, 13
circulatory system, 19–22
Five Element theory, 21, *21*, 24
meridian system, 18
organ system, 13–18 (*see also specific organs*)
self-knowledge via, 23–24
vs. Western Medicine, 8–9
yin and yang, *20*, 20–21, 79, 95, 98, 103–106
Oriental Nutrition, 13
osteoarthritis, 41–42
osteoporosis, 152

pain
arm, 148–149, 157–160
back, 155–156, 159–160
elbow, 157–158
from fibromyalgia, 79–80
finger, 148–149
foot/ankle, 83, 148–149
hand, 148–149
hip, 178–179
joint, 159–160
leg, 148–149, 159–160
neck, 157–158
from nerve damage, 148–149
from scar tissue, 149, 153–154
shoulder, 157–158
toe, 148–149
wrist, 208–209
pancreas. *See* Spleen/Pancreatic system
panic attacks, 39
Parkinson's disease, 161–162
Pericardium, 14, 17

Pituitary gland, 97
pre-menopausal problems. *See* menopausal problems
prostate problems, 173
pulse rates, 51–52, 92–93, 118–119

Qi, 18

reproduction, 105–106, 136–137
restless leg syndrome, 174–175
rheumatoid arthritis, 41–42
Right Thinking, 13
ringing in the ears, 176–177

Sanjiao, 14
scar tissue pain, 149, 153–154
sciatica/hip pain, 178–179
shingles, 180–181
shoulder pain, 157–158
sinus problems, 182–184
skin conditions, 30–31, 185–186
sleep problems. *See also* insomnia
  narcolepsy, 145–147
  snoring, 188–190
Small Intestine, 14
  and constipation, 60–61
  diarrhea due to, 69
  functions, 17, 66
smoking cessation, 187
snoring, 188–190
spinal column
  disk problems, 191–192
  stenosis, 193–194
Spleen/Pancreatic system
  and allergies, 32–34
  and anemia, 36
  and asthma, 43
  and cholesterol, 58
  and diabetes, 64–65
  diarrhea due to, 68
  and fatigue, 77
  and fluid metabolism/distribution, 81
  functions, 16, 66
  hemorrhoids due to, 91
  insomnia due to, 107, 109, 124, 126
  narcolepsy due to, 145
  overview, 14–15
  and sinus problems, 182
  snoring due to, 188–190
Spleen/Pancreatic system (*cont.*)
  varicose veins due to, 205
  and weight problems, 206
Stomach, 14
  and acid reflux/heartburn, 28
  diarrhea due to, 68
  and fatigue, 77
  functions, 17, 66
stress. *See also* Liver
  Bell's Palsy due to, 48
  bodily breakdown due to, 19–20
  difficulty adapting to, 195–197
  and high blood pressure, 51, 92
  TMJ due to, 202
  types, 19
strokes, 171–172
sweating at night, 132–133, 150–151

tendonitis, 198
thyroid imbalances, 96–97, 199–200
TMJ (Temporomandibular Joint) Syndrome, 201–202
toe pain, 148–149
tremors, 203–204

Urinary Bladder, 14, 17
uterus and Endometriosis, 73–74

vaginal dryness, 134–135
varicose veins, 205
vertigo/dizziness, 71–72

water element, 21, *21*, 24
weight problems, 206–207
Western vs. Oriental Medicine, 8–9
wood element, 21, *21*, 24
wrist pain, 208–209. *See also* carpal tunnel syndrome

yin and yang, *20*, 20–21, 79, 95, 98, 103–106